Doctor Morrison's Miracle Guide to Pain-Free Health and Longevity

Marsh Morrison, D.C., Ph.C., F.I.C.C.

Parker Publishing Company, Inc., West Nyack, N.Y.

Library of Congress Cataloging in Publication Data

Morrison, Marsh
    Doctor Morrison's Miracle guide to pain-free
health and longevity.

    Includes index.
    1. Naturopathy. 2. Hygiene. I. Title.
II. Title: Miracle guide to pain-free health
and longevity.
RZ440.M67   615'.535   76-30837
ISBN 0-13-216341-1

This book is dedicated to my great, great five-hundred-generations-ago grandfather,

Adam

. . . whose spark resulted in my being me

*with gratitude and high esteem
because life is such
an ennobling and glorious adventure
when one enjoys nonmedicated, nonsurgicated
Natural Health*

The Effective and Natural Health Benefits of This Book

From the ordinary little common cold to violent migraines or gall bladder attacks or seizures of emphysema—what can you do for them?

There are ways to do things now. Natural methods of self-help that are so remarkably effective as to be unbelievable. To present these natural and very effective methods to you is why this volume was written.

Nowadays we hear the expression, "What's this all about?" I like the expression because it seeks to get into the meaty middle of a matter without wasting time, and this is precisely why it "pleasures me" to tell you at the beginning what this book's all about. It is only fair to do this, and to do it on the very first page. Then if this kind of health information and natural health protection is not what you want, you can turn aside from the book without further waste of time.

It can all be said in a single sentence: *How to be healthy in this unhealthy world*—that's what this book was written to show you, and it *does* show it in every chapter in precise detail.

No matter what you do or don't do about taking care of your health, there are two strikes against you. Two strikes are always and forever working against your health. What are they, these two strikes that imperil your health?

We live in a polluted world. Our substandard ecology is Strike No. One. With every breath we suck gases and toxins into our lungs; this is a drag on our respiratory system. In the following pages I give you simple, sensible and physiologically correct ways to "make do" with the poor oxygen supply that's available to us.

Strike No. Two is gravity, something else that we must face daily. It is a fact that we all live against gravity. Unlike the horizontally-positioned animal, we are not solidly positioned on four legs with our organs in ideal working position. We live straight up and down: *we live against gravity.*

And we suffer such counter-gravity conditions as fallen stomach, drooping eyelids, sagging colon, varicose veins, prolapsed uterus, hernia, hemorrhoids, fallen arches, etc. All this constitutes a drag on our circulatory system. In this book I give you specific corrective programs by which you can sensibly and easily pay the toll that living against gravity exacts from you every day.

Also, this book sets forth in a clear, easy-to-remember way beneficial methods by which your body can quite easily purify your bloodstream and balance your body chemistry. It also shows you how you can relieve your body of pinched nerves wherever they exist in your spinal column, and also how you can siphon off most of the nervous tensions that accumulate within all of us in this rush-rush competitive world. That's what this book's all about.

Those who know my books and lectures are aware that I rebel against drugs for this and that and every other sickness. When those of us with my background and training are in possession of so very many demonstrably *natural* ways to benefit almost every ailment that plagues mankind, how could I do other than rebel against the drugs-for-everything methods?

In this book you will get to know my own research projects, which provide natural health with incredible effectiveness in many cases. Having conducted a variety of research projects, I have gleaned various lessons of importance to health-seeking individuals. But of all my research the single greatest lesson I ever have learned is one that did not revolve around a controlled project, and one that took a half-century to discover. Are you ready for this greatest single discovery I have made? It is this:

When people are educated, it never occurs to them that they may not also be intelligent.

Educated persons imagine that since they have been exposed to the educational processes they are automatically intelligent. Not so. Education is what you know. Intelligence is an analytical matter of how you use what you know, or of having *logical judgment.* Read this again please. Many educated men are not intelligent. Some of the best educated men I have ever known (and had working for me) were unbelievable dunces who lacked simple logical judgment.

Educated people (rather than analytically intelligent) usually insist that their years of study make them importantly knowledgeable—therefore intelligent. But analytical intelligence declares that mere years of study do not guarantee any quality of excellence or usefulness. It depends on what you study, not how long.

That is why I scorn the ordinary drug-giving methods— because they are not scientific. Doctors exclaim indignantly that they are. Well, let us see.

Since the body manufactures its own drugs (chemicals), is it scientific to give drugs from outside? Your organism manufactures all the drug-chemicals it needs, along with its proper nutrition and function. Your body makes insulin, adrenalin, pepsin, cortisone, hormones, hydrochloric acid—everything it needs for its health, growth, and self-repair. Well then, using sheer analytical intelligence rather than being awed by mere education, is it *scientific* to be seeking always and forever new drugs to replace what the body once made but cannot make anymore? Or wouldn't it be actually, honestly, more validly scientific to find out *why* your own body stopped making what it's supposed to make? And, following that, finding out *how* to put the organs back to manufacturing what they were intended to manufacture?

See what happens when we apply the searchlight of analytical intelligence to this business?

It is a physiological fact that your body has what is known as Natural Selectivity. This means that your organism has the intelligent ability to *select* out of what you eat and drink those substances which it *wants* and *needs* and *can use*—rejecting with intelligent selectivity those substances you've swallowed that are incompatible with your body chemistry, those which it knows it doesn't want and cannot use. This is your safeguard and safety valve.

Your individual blood chemistry is as peculiarly your own as your individual fingerprints.

When the food you've consumed gets to the lower part of the intestines, there are little blood-sucking vessels there that suck into your bloodstream *only* that which is appropriate and consonant with your needs, only that which is necessary to and usable by your individual blood chemistry—rejecting all that is not good for you.

I am sure that I have a richer, better, safer and more natural way to health than that made possible by drugs. As you read through this book you will hardly be able to refrain from noting well how sane and relentlessly logical these natural methods are that lead you into natural health.

We know that disease grows increasingly all around us. The word *scientific* betokens a skill, an ability to cope, a know-how in dealing with situations. Our national situation is that almost everyone is ill or ailing to some degree. Human disorder is the order of the day. But the way out of physical disorder into health is not entirely dependent on drugs. There are other methods that use neither drugs nor surgery. These methods are unmistakably set forth in the pages ahead.

Our land is presently awash with more heart disease than ever before. We have more cancer than ever before in the history of the world. We are assailed with more mental illness than in all previous times. There are some 25 million cases of arthritis which drugs and injections cannot reach. There is more diabetes, cerebral palsy, muscular dystrophy, hepatitis, multiple sclerosis, epilepsy, cystic fibrosis, emphysema, renal disease, Parkinson's disease, and even far more common colds than ever before.

In the body of this book I shall devote myself to telling you how to be healthy in an unhealthy world. While showing you how to gain and maintain health, I will fill the ensuing pages with practical and simple and workable natural methods of healing that represent beneficial and practical ways to health.

Your body has a hundred different organs that perform a thousand different functions, all at the same time, with precision and without confusion. While doing this they manufacture and elaborate all the drug-chemicals you need, all the adrenalin and pepsin and cortisone you need merely out of the food you eat, the fluids you drink, and the air you breathe—*provided* you remove the obstructions to self-healing.

The cause of disease is very nearly always obstruction to the flow of healing forces, for the body is a self-healing organism. Since medicines suppress symptoms they are exactly, I think, what one must *avoid* to get well. Once the obstructing interferences have left the body, it is in a state of ease. Until then it is in a state of dis-ease.

The human bloodstream, as indicated previously, does not accept just anything into itself, for it has the faculty of Natural Selectivity which permits it to choose what it needs, and wants, and can use in its own blood chemistry, rejecting all else through the four avenues of elimination: kidneys, bowels, exhalation and skin.

The heart is usually overworked and overstrained after receiving a jolting infusion of a foreign toxic agent (a shot) into the blood which that heart needs to pump around. It wears out earlier and gets sick under such strain and overwork. Result: an increase in heart disease attributable, I fully believe, to the increased giving of "shots."

The kidneys are forever overstrained in filtering out the residue of the waste product of these toxic shots, and they get sick from such needless overwork and overstrain. Result: an alarming increase in renal degenerative diseases since the increased shot-giving vogue. It is physiologically possible that some of the unacceptable, unmetabolized protein products of the foreign-injected agent tend to have an affinity for attaching themselves to brain tissue—like barnacles on a ship—and there has been a shattering increase in mental illness since the drug-and-shot increases came into being.

It is not for nothing that I have titled this book *MIRACLE GUIDE TO PAIN-FREE HEALTH AND LONGEVITY.* The methods presented in these pages are precisely programmed to achieve freedom from pain and to gain a longer-than-usual life span.

Here I set forth the ways and natural methods by which almost everyone (barring those with far-advanced, irreversible pathologies) can gain and maintain health.

Here I set forth those enormously valuable drills for restoring and resting the eyes, for when you rest the eyes you rest the entire body.

Do you hope for a diet that will tend to strengthen the weak heart? A diet to normalize badly functioning kidneys? To improve the breathing apparatus and help such respiratory ailments as emphysema and asthma? A diet that works toward balancing the body chemistry, or a diet that often completely helps migraines and other headache syndromes? Even a *nondiet-like* diet for urinary disturbances and bladder weaknesses? All these are presented in this book. Also—note this—a compromised diet for those who feel they can't follow diets.

All of the aforementioned are given herein in simplicity and detail. That's the kind of book this is.

As a writer and a doctor I have no axe to grind, none except truth. I deeply want to help those millions of lost and frightened sick in the land to find health. If any other method did the job I'd gladly become a disciple of such a method. But I see no hope for the world of sick people in finding more and more drugs, rather in finding techniques by which the body can put its own organs back to their natural job of making the drugs they were created to make: insulin, adrenalin, cortisone, pepsin, hydrochloric acid, hormones, etc. My goal, and the chief goal of this book, is to set forth techniques which bypass the need for surgery and lead you into pain-free health and longevity.

I have written this long introduction purposely, for in these pages I wish to give you all the "reasons why" of the book so that the remaining pages will be left free for pragmatic, workable, how-to-get-well drills and techniques and advices. In this introduction you learn why this book was necessary and why one must set up natural techniques and programs calculated to remove bodily obstructions in order to get back his health and then maintain it. With such explanations and philosophies out of the way, now we can devote the book proper to the practical business of showing you all the methods by which to attain and maintain good solid, dependable *natural* health.

So, again, you can see and know what this book is all about.

Marsh Morrison, D.C., Ph.C., F.I.C.C.
Cottage Grove, Oregon

Contents

Chapter Seven: THE QUESTION OF THE COLD PLUNGE .. 47

Why cold baths and especially "the cold plunge" may be a neurological shock despite the tingling warmth one experiences afterward.

Chapter Eight: A DISCOVERY IN BREAST SELF-EXAMINATION **51**

Vital research in the field of lumps in the female breast. How women can transilluminate their own suspicious areas and discover their own tumors—and how to get the body to "eat them up" in a safe, physiologically natural way.

Chapter Nine: CHEWING AND DIGESTION **55**

Exploring why gum-chewing persons so often chew their way into digestive problems. Why it may not be true that chewing gum "aids digestion," but too often creates indigestion.

Chapter Ten: DANGER IN THE BATHROOM **59**

A research adventure with toothbrushes. Since bathrooms frequently have foul odors remaining after bowel evacuations, should our toothbrushes hang where smelly bacteria can enter their bristles? And should towels also be exposed to such bacteria? We rub the bacteria-laden toothbrush bristles into our gums, and the bacteria-filled towels into our eyes, so shouldn't they be hung away from the foulness, *inside* a cabinet?

Chapter Eleven: A SIMPLE AID FOR ARTERIOSCLEROSIS AND THE ELDERLY **63**

An entirely new and arresting look into the way we usually rest on our backs, often piled high on a few pillows "for comfort." Boosting up the elderly and the sick especially may be entirely wrong because it forces circulation to work uphill, against gravity. The sick already suffer from circulatory lacks in many cases. The elderly almost always suffer from a cranial oxygen lack, so this whole "customary" method needs a serious reappraisal.

Chapter Twelve: AVOIDING DYSPEPSIA AND THE DOWAGER'S HUMP **67**

A very informative research project into the connection between a stoop-shouldered (rounded spine) condition and stomach trouble. How a forward-bent or kyphotic spine may pinch nerves that conduct functional power to the digestive organs. This chapter presents a valuable specific body movement that tends to unpinch such compressed nerves.

A disturbing investigation of the harm that can be caused by one-sided exercises. Why the various sports that use only one side of the body to the exclusion of the other should be avoided in certain conditions. The superiority of rowing, bicycling, walking, and other two-sided activities over unilateral sports such as bowling, tennis, golf. How unilateral exercises and sports can set up sciatica and even bilateral strains.

Reassessing the value or harmfulness of the after-dinner stroll. Animals romp before a meal but nap after eating. The blood should be in the digestive organs following your meal, not pulled away into the walking muscles.

A new researching look at the common cold. Why a cure is impossible; it is a waste of time to be seeking a cure for the cold because the cold itself is the cure. When the body is loaded with toxic debris beyond continued endurance, it reflexively starts up the symptoms of a cold and the waste products are burned up with a fever or coughed up or sneezed out, etc.

Rethinking the matter of sunbathing. . .when it is good and when harmful. How you can judge the safe and noncancer-causing time by the shadow you cast in the sun.

Astonishing new research findings in the field of high protein consumption. How the body is rigidly limited in its capacity to utilize protein and why an overuse putrefies into smelly acids that give human stool matter a foul odor not chacteristic of the stools of low-protein-eating animals.

A researcher puts the right end of the telescope on fruit skins: to eat or not to eat? The human body may not have the enzymes to fully digest skins, which is one reason why we find undigested tomato skins in the stools.

A researcher discovers the best time to exercise, and when you may expect greatest benefits from specific body movements. What you gain at bedtime you retain during bedtime.

A valuable discovery—why even good foods do not necessarily translate into good health. The potential value of any food is not its actual value. Why this is so, and what must be done.

Adventuring into the relative values of upright exercises and horizontal exercises. Why the benefits are greater when the heart does not need to pump blood upward, straight against gravity.

A restudy of milk as a human food. Milk is chiefly a protein, and proteins were meant to be chewed, never drunk. Is this why pediatricians keep busy with infant problems, changing their formulas and watering down their milk consumption with more physiologically compatible fare?

A researching adventure into a safe haven for almost all sick persons—The Primate Diet. Man is a primate and fruit is (or was originally) his natural food. Why it is that when baffled about your condition, or when the doctor is baffled about it, this diet is safe and beneficial in most cases.

Encouraging researches into heart-building drills for cardiac sufferers. Specific ways to stimulate the development of auxiliary little arteries in stricken parts of the heart. How such newly formed arteries can feed the damaged portions of the heart in coronary occlusion.

A dramatic study of how to expand the memory and cause new brain cells to pop into activity—the way Aristotle employed the method. By fantasizing geometric patterns and figures such as circles and squares and triangles, you can nourish the brain cells and enliven the thinking processes.

An awakening research into how to strengthen the breathing apparatus. Techniques for giving new power to the diaphragm, vigor that specifically aids asthma, emphysema, bronchial troubles. Count twice as long exhaling as inhaling to invigorate breathing muscles. Widen the ribs through side-to-side separation. Raise the arms and pant to give resonance to the voice.

A valuable reappraisal that ensures newer, better and more natural health—the chemical cause of disease versus the mechanical cause. We are born with a complete chemical factory; at birth the body was able to manufacture adrenalin, insulin, hormones, cortisone, pepsin, and everything else. We were not born with adequate mechanical equipment; in infancy we could not even sit up, much less stand, balance, run, heave, lug, tug, strain. In adjusting to the demands of straight-up, two-legged contra-gravity living, the body is jarred or strained out of mechanical adjustment, and no machine that is out of adjustment can function normally. A rememberable lesson in how faulty body mechanics can disrupt normal body chemistry, but not the other way around.

Remarkable techniques for determining and correcting one's own nerve pressures in the neck. Self-tests by which anyone can tell if there are pinched nerves in the neck area, and how to unpinch them quite easily.

Researching some quite pleasant and natural ways to improve the eyes. Humans do all their work with eyes straight front, and this pulls eyeballs from their round shape. These drills can exercise the peripheral muscles and bring eyes back to their normal "roundness," with resulting improvement in function. A technique that often reaches headaches (migraine) successfully and naturally.

Diets for all seasons and conditions. Specific self-help programs for the following:

> Losing weight naturally
> Strengthening a weak heart
> Normalizing kidneys and bladder
> Helping asthma and emphysema naturally
> Aiding gallstone conditions
> Balancing your blood chemistry
> Reaching your migraines and other headaches
> Soothing and nourishing your nervous system
> PLUS—a compromise diet if you are one of
>   those who feel they can't follow diets.

The best exercises for pain-free longevity. Self-help methods for treating joints, muscles, ligaments, and organs to relieve pain. Entirely natural and correct techniques that tend to give your body flexibility and a younger appearance.

Putting the whole book together. All the self-help methods and techniques of the book, plus all the drills and natural aids, finally concentrated into nutshell sentences for quick ready reference and easy recall.

Chapter One

A Discovery
About the Drinking of Fluids

Do you suffer from urinary problems such as night rising, or excessive voiding, or even dribbling?

I recall running into a method that benefits this, and it was almost by accident. The method was simplicity itself. I merely stopped, and changed, the drinking habits of patients who had such problems. For a time, perhaps no longer than two weeks, they were prohibited from drinking soups, coffee, tea, water, soft drinks or any kinds of liquid items whatever.

By a kind of accident I had discovered that most people were overfluidizing themselves. They were pouring too much liquid stuff into their innards. They guzzled water and other fluids just like pouring water down a car radiator. This caused the inner conditions that I had discovered (which I will explain presently), so for the duration of this research project I cut off their fluid supply. They were advised to obtain all their liquids only from the pure natural juices within tomatoes, apples, peaches, grapes and the various vegetables and other foodstuffs that they consumed daily.

And what do you suppose happened? Almost all of them reported a lessening in night rising, then no night rising at all. Those who had trouble retaining their urine found they had no need to make a mad dash for the nearest toilet lest they dribble and wet their underthings. And those with insomnia found this a blessing. The business of getting up at night and breaking up their sleep—this in most cases was a business that diminished and finally evaporated.

I can hear the reader saying, almost incredulously, *but why?* No fluid intake at all? Why?

Well, thereby hangs the tale.

Do We Drink Only When Thirsty?

People wake up in the morning and immediately reach for their coffee. One day it occurred to me that the purpose of drinking is to fill a physiological need. Any kind of drink should be only in answer to a thirst signal. If this is true—and it is certainly *physiologically* true—does anyone awake with a thirst for coffee? Or for tea or juice or whatever? Or is it that drinking has become merely a habit—a sign of our culture and our times?

It would be easy to find out if this track I was on had any merit. Several of the patients in my busy clinic had trouble with urination. They urinated too often, or when voiding their urine, it burned, smarted or irritated them. Some couldn't hold urine any length of time at all. Others had to run like mad to make it to the toilet and then found they had precious little to excrete. Most of them had to rise several times a night, and a few even suffered the embarrassment of dribbling.

Just then I happened to be invited to a cocktail party and on entering I was asked, "What are you drinking?" I noted that everyone else was asked the same thing. In our social scheme hardly anything goes on without drinking. But were people thirsty for a drink? Were they thirsty for any kind of drink any more than they arose thirsty for coffee? If not, anything they drank definitely was not filling a physiological need in their bodies and perhaps did harm to their urinary apparatus.

I decided I could run a little research project among those patients in the office who had urinary complaints.

Accordingly, I asked my office assistants to go through the files and pick out 20 patients with bladder or kidney difficulties. These I separated into two groups. The first group was allowed to continue in the old way, and the other ten were disallowed any fluids whatever aside from what came naturally in their fruits, vegetables, meats and so forth.

"The best possible water," I explained to them, "is the natural, unchlorinated and untreated kind that you can get in a peach or a pineapple, an orange or a watermelon, a stalk of celery, a ripe tomato or a zucchini squash. That wonderful fluid has been refined and purified in nature's laboratory. That's the only fluid you will take on board for the next fortnight. No water, soft drinks, beer, soup, coffee or tea, etc."

There was one more thing I told them: "Never drink even orange juice or tomato juice in a big, guzzling draught. Sip your fluids; don't pour them down your gullet like water into your radiator tank."

I told them to be utterly serious about this experiment and to report the results in seven days. They did. What they reported is what triggered this little chapter on the kidneys and bladder as related to the nearly universal overdrinking of fluids by human beings.

No Drinks . . . No Night Rising

This was the first of many similar research projects in the area of overdrinking. It all really began when I was yet a student. I was in the dissection class, and the cadaver before me was that of an elderly man. I remember comparing the tissue of the corpse I was working on with a piece of lean animal beefsteak.

The butcher shop steak was dry; by comparison it was unbelievably dry. The slab of human muscle meat I held in my hand was wet. The cells of the tissue appeared waterlogged; they were bathed in fluid. The cells also were drowned in what seemed to be uncirculating lymph.

It occurred to me that the cells thus drowned in fluid could not possibly function as well as cells not bathed in needless liquid masses. Although I was almost a doctor already, I was still too young at the business to relate it to anything of significance. I was not yet enough of a doctor to have it make sense.

Later this early impression returned to nibble at my mind, and it was this that began my research in overdrinking. I already had been in practice almost a decade and had gone back for some postgraduate study. In the dissection laboratory I recognized with shock that the man on the slab was one I had known casually in life as a desert rat, one with an insatiable lust for gold who'd spent most of his adult years in solitude in the sandy regions of Arizona.

Unlike the flesh of most people, this man's muscle tissue was not sopping wet with unneeded fluid. He had died in a cave-in accident, with his skull crushed like an eggshell. But the years of unquenched thirst while packing his gear across sun-soaked deserts showed in his tissues. The man's vital organs were in good shape. They were almost untouched by age. The privations of the years—especially being deprived of fluids—had contributed to a good organism and had given him a quality of health not often equalled by men who drank all the fluids they ever wanted.

The need for serious research in this area asserted itself. Later I was to learn that almost everyone overdrank, that most night rising could be stopped by stopping overdrinking and that a large body of symptomatology now attributed to the urinary bladder and kidneys could be made to disappear when overdrinking disappeared. I had learned what was in a way an earth-shaking, incredible truth. It was a truth that demanded a complete rethink of our human drinking patterns. These patterns did not relate to alcoholic drinking but to the drinking of plain water, soda, beer, soups, milk, coffee, tea or anything at all.

Are We All Overdrinkers?

With almost no exceptions we indeed are overdrinkers. Our drinking is out of habit or out of social, time-passing amenities. At any social gathering, as previously noted, the recurring phrase is, "What are you drinking?" This culture of ours has evolved in such a way that we hardly know how to preserve protocol or have any gathering without serving drinks. My acquaintance, the desert rat, had hardly drunk anything at all in his entire life, and he enjoyed health in his vital organs. Even when he'd come to town and treated himself to a whiskey, he never drank it in the usual sense; he sipped it. He never guzzled or quaffed anything. His throat was never a funnel leading to an inner storage tank.

We are indeed all overdrinkers. The studies I conducted with groups under correct research controls and strict supervision taught me several arresting truths. With the force of a sledgehammer blow, I learned that we must drink only in answer to thirst just as we must eat only in answer to hunger. And I learned that people who suffered from ailments or functional symptoms related to the bladder or kidneys almost uniformly improved when told not to drink tea or coffee or *anything* simply because it's breakfast, coffeebreak time or tea time as in England.

Whatever Anyone Drinks Must Be in Answer to a Thirst Signal

If you ever drink anything at all that is not in answer to an actual thirst within you or to still a desire for a thirst-quenching fluid, what you drink can harm you. It does not fill a real need, is not physiologically desirable and is potentially damaging. If continued, this in my opinion can be violently inimical to bodily cellular health.

Later studies revealed to me that underdrinkers, rather than overdrinkers, were among the healthiest humans on earth. Most long-lived inhabitants of this planet drank sparingly of fluids. Moreover, they never swilled but took their drinks by sips, drop by drop, not poured down in rivulets.

Back to that cadaver of student days. He was elderly. He had spent his life overdrinking, and his tissues showed it. In subsequent observations almost the identical pattern appeared in elderly men and women. When I related the observations I'd made on that cadaver as a student to my findings in strict research projects afterward I learned something I profoundly want the readers of these pages to know. It is this: If you are like other overdrinkers of our society, and if you are plagued by night rising or urinary problems, a very large but so-far incalculable part of your maladies can probably be attributed to that lifelong habit of drinking too many fluids, especially of guzzling rather than sipping them.

What You Ought to Do Beginning Tomorrow

I now ask you to read and consider this carefully. You will rise tomorrow morning and reach for your morning coffee. When you do, ask yourself whether you have a thirst for coffee. Will you have a thirst for anything? If not, you are abusing your inner plumbing mechanism by filling it with fluids not physiologically needed by that organism of yours. If, however, you do have an actual thirst, try making a pinhole in an orange or ripe tomato and sucking out the fluid drop by drop. Just note if that doesn't quench your thirst beyond anything you ever imagined.

During the day, beginning tomorrow, resolve not to swill any fluids of any kind and forego the consumption of soup, milk, water or beverages. Chew every mouthful so thoroughly that it will self-liquidize merely by insalivation. Do this for a single week as a test and note the difference in your energy level, your weight, your changed pattern of night rising and the way your weight is changed by redistribution of bodily masses into the right rather than the wrong places.

Please learn to listen to what I call "the wisdom of the body." Be on the alert for a thirst signal, and for what is not that at all but something that has become a silly, ruinous social compulsion.

When my patients in control groups began to see this "wisdom of the body" they proceeded to improve almost magically in nearly every way, in many cases not merely improving but getting well entirely just because they stopped taking unneeded water, soft drinks or beverages into their bodies.

The elderly patients with urinary incontinence and even dribbling difficulties were especially grateful. Many were mentally relieved also when they lost their terrible hurry to reach a bathroom lest they void in their clothing. And the chronic insomniacs felt twice-blessed. Now they could sleep through the night without dancing to the toilet several times per session and needing to fight themselves back to sleep after each toilet trip.

PUTTING IT ALL TOGETHER

People with insomnia improved in many ways just because of the single benefit of a night's sleep without interruption. All this stemmed merely from not overdrinking. Here was an area that to my knowledge had never been researched. Why not? What field was there that had greater importance than urinary difficulties, bladder problems, sleeplessness and its consequences?

Having learned that people overdrank fluids of all kinds, I did not consider this a vastly earth-shaking discovery in itself. But in putting together the benefits in human health that led from this I came face to face with ancillary projects of far-reaching significance. I believe the word for it is concatenation. The concatenation, or chain-like linkage to other investigations, provided me with a new skill in the case management of various serious kidney ailments and urinary bladder dysfunctions.

It all had a jolting effect on people in the clinic. We became convinced that 1) everyone drank too much, and 2) thereby overworked their kidneys. We felt sure that the best and easiest way to provide human kidneys with the rest that they almost always very much needed was just to stop loading the body with liquids. This was metabolically the kindest way to rest those many hundreds of overworking uriniferous tabules; and since the human body always tends toward the normal (note how your cuts and bruises mend normally), with a proper physiological rest the damages in kidneys tended to self-heal and self-repair.

When all this was put together for patients they came up with one worry. If they took all their fluids solely from an occasional tomato or piece of fruit, would they not run the risk of becoming dehydrated? I had to assure them that dehydration was a largely unresearched, usually fluffy medical statistic. In forty years of dealing with thousands of patients I could recall only one identifiable case of true dehydration. Therefore I caution the reader to take himself in hand and, say for a week or two, resist all such health-ruining temptations. You cannot hurt anything by a mere week or two of this. And you just possibly might reach what has been unreachable in your illness charts.

Final Note

Beginning tomorrow, and without fail, for your own health's sake ask yourself this question: Is any of this bladder or kidney trouble, or is any of the rising incidence of heart and brain and lung and many other diseases in any way due to our unceasingly rising overdrinking habits?

And starting tomorrow, for sure, do not drink anything that is not triggered by thirst. No water, especially. Get your best, purest water out of a tomato or juicy peach, pear, melon, persimmon, grapes, etc. And swallow the juice slowly. Try it for a week. In a mere, single week you may discover that ailments you were resigned to enduring all your life have gone, left you, fairly evaporated away.

Chapter Two

Avoiding the Danger of Hot Foods

Do you occasionally find yourself in a state of fright because of hoarseness?

Some cancerologists warn that if hoarseness recurs or persists it can be a sign of cancer.

Is your hoarseness a persistent thing? And when it clears up for a time, does it tend to come back? And do you at the same time embarrassingly belch or regurgitate your food?

In this chapter I want to explain how such symptoms can be caused merely by the act of drinking fluids that are so hot that you can't dip your fingers into them. Hot coffee, for example. Or hot soup. The delicate membrane that lines your throat—and your mouth, lips, esophagus—gets irritated and even blistered when it is contacted by very hot liquid. And when nature fights off these daily insults to your tissues, the result is often a state of hoarseness.

The fact is that even such serious states as cancer of the throat, mouth and esophagus have been alleviated and also eliminated with the elimination of hot foods and drinks. When I ordered patients to stop eating hot foods and drinking anything they couldn't touch with the bare hand, they began to improve.

In this chapter I also wish to discuss the matter of belching and other digestive ills.

It is interesting and helpful to know how all of this came about.

***

Researching the "Hotness" of Foods

I was in a restaurant, having a heated discussion with an acquaintance, another doctor—a medical doctor. As my eyes were fixed on the man across the table, and I was talking my head off about the new techniques for rebuilding a blood flow to the heart, my hand reached automatically to the cigarette pack at my side, for in those foolish days I smoked the abominable "coffin nails." The cigarettes were beside my coffee cup. My eyes were unwaveringly on the doctor as I spoke. As my hand swept to the side for the cigarettes the fingers landed instead inside the coffee cup.

"Ouch!" My fingers came out in a hurry. Why hadn't I the sense to look where I was placing my hand, instead of looking at the doctor while I reached for the cigarettes? But it was not all in vain. The event triggered a piece of research that later helped a lot of patients. Thus—accidentally—are some research projects born.

While nursing the burned fingers, especially the right forefinger which I used a lot in my work, the wheels inside my head began spinning. That coffee was too hot for my fingers, yet I poured it down my throat every day, several times a day. My forefinger is toughened. It is protected by a 2-layered envelope of skin that is further subdivided into six protective layers, yet it couldn't stand the heat that the thin, delicate mucosa of my esophagus was forced to stand daily. If my hardened, tough finger got burned with just a second of contact with hot coffee, what happened in the gullet during the several seconds it took the coffee to traverse the tube and enter the stomach?

I was onto something! Another adventure in research. It took several days for the burn to be assuaged in the fingers. I wouldn't dream of dipping those fingers into another cup of hot fluid while they were still healing. But what about my poor esophagus?

My knowledge of physiology took over. Every time I drank coffee or tea or hot soup the membrane lining in my tube to the stomach got burned, scalded, blistered. It couldn't be otherwise— the mucosa was so very delicate and tender. Did I wait to give it a chance to heal, as I did my finger? No! In another few hours I would drink another cup of hot coffee or similar insult. Before the mucous membrane had a chance to get "unblistered" from the burning contact of the last cup I'd subject it to a new burn. And this would go on. On and on, and on and on.

Can You Tolerate Immersing Your Fingers into What You Drink?

I remember speaking about this matter to my young office assistant, Dr. Joyce Flaherty, a newly graduated chiropractic doctor who was already a brilliant investigator. "Make me a list of all on your treatment schedule who have husky or peculiar voices," I requested.

"Those with whiskey tenor voices?" he smiled.

"The same," I said. "I'll gather up mine and bring all of them in for a lecture one evening soon."

All our office patients with hoarse, rather than diaphragmatic voices were advised most strictly to forego the use of hot fluids—*all* hot ingestive items. At the time we were seeing some 60 to 70 patients daily in our busy clinic, and thus had plenty of research material at hand.

Without exception every patient reported a greater sense of well-being. Voices became de-hoarsed, vibrant, clear. A few with belching and regurgitation complaints reported an end to their distresses. With this one smallish piece of original research we were helping a lot of sick persons who were lost and frightened and hadn't until then known where to turn for help. They dropped their medicines and grandmother remedies. All they did was remove the obstruction to healing, as we so often called it; that is, they stopped irritating the body in such a way so as to make health impossible.

"Nature cures, and the doctor pockets the fee," I would often say to my patients, quoting Ben Franklin. "The body tends toward the normal. It wants to be well and stay well. If you have a cut hand or a rash, these things get well without even awaiting a doctor's diagnosis. Just remove the blockages or obstructions to healing, and the body will heal itself."

To me, doctor means teacher. I took this seriously, forever teaching patients the rules of "healthifying" the body.

"I may be baffled by your condition," I'd explain, "but the body never is. The body knows what's the matter, and it knows how to heal and mend and repair whatever is the matter. *Healing is an inside job.* All we have to do is prepare the conditions that make healing possible. No suppressing drugs . . . Sufficient nerve supply . . . Compatible foods . . . Proper exercise and oxygenation . . . *And no hot fluids or foods.*"

PUTTING IT ALL TOGETHER

Do not allow yourself to swallow any beverage that is too hot to dip your fingers into. Do not eat any food that you cannot hold between your thumb and forefinger for a few minutes. Avoid any food item that burns your tongue or lips or mouth. This is an absolute rule. Without observing it you cannot *reasonably* expect to enjoy optimum health.

Chapter Three

On Using Electric Blankets

Do you suffer from cold hands and feet? Even though the rest of your body is warm, do people say that your extremities are ice-cold when they touch them?

If you use one of those nice cozy electric blankets, you may be in for a shock. I do not mean an electric shock. The shocker is that the artificial heat fed into the body may be causing your body to quit generating its own heat the way it is supposed to.

Not all cold extremities, of course, are due to this. But many of them, I have discovered, either are caused or helped along by the employment of an unnatural producer of heat when your body was intended and created to produce its own.

When something that your own body should be doing is steadily done *for* it, then a strange thing occurs. The body loses those functions that it does not employ. If you take away the body's need to generate heat throughout the night and get an electric blanket to do the job instead, then watch out. The body, in that case, tends to give up the work of manufacturing heat— why should it do so when something artificial is doing the job for it?—and then the person in this state tends to feel more cold when not in contact with the artificial "heat-giver," the electric blanket.

As I have written before, even when the use of electric blankets is not the cause of cold hands and feet, in most cases where I discovered other causes the use of these blankets also contributed to the trouble.

It was strange how all this came to my notice.

***

Adventuring into Electric Blankets

The muscular young man came into the clinic complaining of cold hands and feet. The elderly couple came in saying they both suffered from cold extremities. In the course of giving her history the lady said an arresting thing.

"I can't see why we should be this way, Doctor Morrison. We bought those new electric blankets and are both as comfy as bugs in rugs all night. Yet we shiver all day."

The sentence of the lady clicked. They were comfortable all night by reason of electrically generated heat, not heat created in their own bodies.

I was at that time reading a voluminous and very popular book, *Gone With the Wind.* Every evening, after a hard day at the office, I also snuggled into one of those newly advertised electric blankets. For ten long evenings I'd read the exciting novel to the end, snug in my electric blanket and stupidly permitting an artificial contraption to be generating heat that the body alone should be manufacturing. And I too was noticing the first signs of cold distal extremities.

It triggered an adventure in research. I questioned every patient, particularly those who complained of debilitated states and cold feet, cold fingertips and so on. Suddenly I had to know how many were using electric blankets to provide body warmth.

A good, dependable rule in physiology kept bothering me. *What you don't use, you lose,* It's a way of saying that nature takes away those functions that we do not employ. One mustn't allow something on the outside to provide heat that the body itself was intended to provide. Just start depending on an electric blanket to generate your inner heat and your body's own thermogenic centers will lie down on the job and quit performing. So let's put the rule down again: What we don't use, we lose.

In nearly every case under this fabulously revealing research observation, X-rays and the usual workup showed nothing wrong to warrant those cold hands and feet. So it had to be blamable on those new, delicious, tempting electric blankets.

I didn't order the patients to discard the blankets. Of course not! They were still very fine aids if properly used, and they were still useful as blankets.

PUTTING IT ALL TOGETHER

Use your electric blankets merely as warmup contraptions before going to bed. Getting into bed between cold sheets is still a kind of neurological shock. It's a shock better avoided. So the electric blanket should be used to make the sheets toast-warm for ten to fifteen minutes before retiring. Then, once inside the warm bed, the electricity should be turned off. Thereafter the blanket serves as just that—merely a blanket or coverlet. All through the night your own body must generate the heat needed for the slowed-down metabolic processes of the restorative sleep time.

Chapter Four

Resting in Bed Properly

Do you awaken most mornings feeling just as tired as when you went to sleep? Do you occasionally feel giddy, a little lightheaded, with the sensation that you did not have enough blood flowing through your brain?

It may be that you are right.

It is in the blood, you know, that oxygen is carried to the brain. If not properly oxygenated, the feeling can indeed be that of giddiness or lightheadedness. And this can also bring on memory lapses. I refer to the forgetfulness that bothers many oldsters, but which also embarrasses younger people from time to time.

Any or all of the foregoing symptoms easily may be caused by an insufficient flow of blood to the head. This is so because we live against gravity. And they are also caused by a low grade of nutritional interchange in the cranium—which, you may be surprised, is often the result of our sleeping on our backs.

Just try something new for a week, or maybe two or three. Get into a kind of knee-chest resting position for 5-minute stretches twice a day. This means that you maintain your weight on your knees and elbows so that the chest is lower than the hips. This will reverse gravity and assuredly can benefit you. Of equal importance for a week or fortnight, avoid sleeping on your back altogether. And certainly avoid boosting yourself up high on pillows, for it is harder for the blood to flow to the brain uphill.

Is this clear? Does it make sense? You can see that it may benefit you enormously and can hardly do you harm to try it.

A Rethink into Bed Rest on One's Back

I had been watching television in my part-time home deep inside the interior of Mexico. A Mexican dairy firm was boasting about their cleanliness in milk production and I decided to drive out and see. People were saying they were not sanitary at all. As a scientist I had to know for myself, not depend on what people "were saying."

While at the dairy I observed some cows at rest. They were lying down on their legs, their forelegs turned under them. In this position their vital thoracic and abdominal organs were free to function without restraint. It came to me with the thrill of discovery that that's not a benefit enjoyed by human beings at all.

I recalled that all the cattle I'd ever seen that did not rest standing up on their four legs never lay on their backs when lying down. They preferred to lie on their sides. On the back their organs would in a sense be working upside down. Instead of being free to function in an unhampered way the organs would be lying against the backbone. They would be compressed, kind of flattened in the rear, needing to operate against the hardness of bone in contact with the softness of functioning tissue.

This caused me to go back to first principles in physiology. The human body is not unlike that of the animal body. From the spinal configurations it is pretty clear that the human body would function best in a horizontal state. In the straight up-and-down state that humans operate in, the heart works uphill against gravity, veins dilate for the same reason, we breathe with the apex of each lung instead of with the lower lobes because the diaphragm flops into wrong "situs" in the vertical position. Besides, man suffers from a host of contragravity conditions: fallen stomach, drooping eyelids, varicose veins, prolapsed uterus, hemorrhoids, hernia, sagging colon, fallen arches, etc.

In the horizontal state, on our hands and knees for example, the heart and lungs and abdominal viscera would be functioning in a free, unhampered state. But if we rolled backward onto the spine these organs would be operating upside-down, against gravity in a way, and be hampered by flopping backward against the vertebral column.

This was truly a revelation. It constituted a rethink that had all the earmarks of a major research project. But when I brought it to my colleagues, a bit diffidently I suppose, because of the immensity of its possibilities and newness of the concept, I was met almost with dismissal and scorn.

"Since time immemorial man has rested best on his back," said one. "Are you thinking of redesigning all the beds in the world?" suggested another.

Is a Stupid Thing Smart Because Millions Do It?

Nevertheless, I did studies in dissection and performed tests upon volunteers. These people were instructed to rest lying face down on a curved couch which I'd devised to let their organs hang loose. From these I feel sure that there is a need for one of those "agonizing reappraisals" in the field of human rest.

How Should Sick People Get Their Rest?

How should a sick or debilitated person really rest? Just because the manner of doing it has always been flat on one's back does not make it positively the best way. Observations in dissections show at times an unaccountable flatness, or bone ridges, on the posterior aspect of the liver, for example. This may be because the very large liver—a gland, really, with one-third of the body's blood in it at all times—operates to its disadvantage during a third of its life, the hours while in bed lying on the back.

I am of the belief that beds and mattresses should be differently designed. One day I mean to contact bedding manufacturers and show them a plan for perfect and physiologically proper bed rest on mattresses that allow human organs to hang loose and free instead of hampering their function.

Meanwhile, for those who must have *meanwhile* help, read and heed what follows.

PUTTING IT ALL TOGETHER

Try to lie on your side rather than on your back. Either the left or right side; the heart is not so far over to the left of the body as to interfere with cardiac function. For perfect resting time, as a present to your organs, lie on your knees and elbows with your head overhanging the edge of the bed. This puts the head a bit lower than the body, a fine position for cranial reoxygenation at the same time. Do this for a few minutes whenever you can during the day or evening. If you can construct it, make a split-headpiece breathing space for your nose in the mattress, and also a dished-out area for the female breasts so as to remove binding constrictions anywhere, then rest face downward in bed. This I believe is the mattress of the future. If pillows are at the same time placed under the abdomen to round out the spine, it's a further help to easy metabolic processes. With a rounded-out vertebral column there is a separation of spinal discs, and more space for the flow of nutrition through the vertebral arteries plus better nerve supply through the nerve pathways.

Chapter Five

On Constipation Difficulties

If constipation is a constant worry and affliction in your life, what follows will amaze you and probably benefit you beyond belief.

If you're "hooked" on enemas, **or** what are euphemistically called high colonic irrigations, I urge you to read on.

Some people who get into the enema habit become so dependent thereafter that they just cannot have a bowel evacuation without artificially washing out their bottom. And this may all be needless.

One possible way out is to squat while at stool. When a human being squats doing his BM—the way our forefathers did in the backwoods before the days of toilets—something very natural and helpful happens. In the squatting position the lower bowel tends to open out or lengthen in size, thus permitting the passage of stool more easily and naturally.

If you who read this are a pregnant woman with the daily problem of constipation ever since you became pregnant—well, this all came about because of a very pregnant young lady who was also very constipated.

***

Researching Adventures in BMs, Enemas and Toilet Bowls

The young, vibrant woman was supremely happy in her pregnancy. But she had a single, small complaint. She was constipated. Before the onset of her pregnancy she had never had this trouble. Now the great worry was that fecal retention might affect the baby.

The case history and examination revealed no reason for the problem. I hated doing barium X-rays and suchlike; even in those days some 25 years ago I'd written and lectured against radiographs because of the carcinogens—they could be cancer-causing. And those disarming but imponderable rays could abort a pregnancy.

What I decided upon was what is called a bimanual "weighing" examination. My exploring finger in the rectum told me that the enlarged womb was making a kind of dent into the rectal walls. It was a mechanical thing. The uterus, being already quite large, was pressing into the rectum and making the tube small, thus preventing the downward passage of stool matter. I merely told the young woman to bend far forward while she was at stool, explaining that this would probably cause a forward movement or shifting of the womb and clear the rectum.

Eureka! It was all she needed and the lady was happy. She had gone to another doctor who advised enemas, but these worked only in an on-and-off way. Her aunt was a satisfied patient at the office and she came to "try" me. Early on I explained that I could not ordinarily abide enemas, which pleased her. The human colon is a self-cleansing tube and in my opinion should not be tampered with or artificially cleansed, any more than the human nose, having mucus and cilia to keep it automatically clean, needs nose drops and such drugstore items.

Another thing, while I'm lowering the boom on enemas, they tend to balloon out the lower part of the rectum. People who take enemas with frequency, and especially if they follow the foolish advice to retain as much water for as long as they can hold it, develop a pouch-like area in the lower rectum where fecal matter can accumulate. Barium studies show this clearly. Enemas should therefore be avoided—which goes double for high colonic washings.

The ease with which the pregnant woman overcame her

constipation problem caused research wheels to start revolving in my head. All she needed to do was lean forward enough to take the weight and pressure of the gravid womb off her rectum. Then there was no obstruction to evacuating the bowel. It was a mechanical problem, yet one for which harmful chemical ingredients such as phenolphthalein are prescribed.

Tip Toilet Seats Up in Front

This adventure in research led me back to oldtime, pre-toilet days. When people needed to defecate they went behind the bushes and squatted. In squatting, something happened that was physiologically perfect. The descending colon and the rectum both elongated properly, which permitted a thorough passage of the stools.

I recalled early student days in Paris and other places in Europe. In many restaurants they had granite or marble slabs alongside a wide trough, and into these stone slabs were indented footprints where one placed his shoes and squatted. On a later trip I asked about the incidence of constipation in such places. Despite the overuse of rich foods and constipating pastries common in European capitals, constipation was less current there than here.

The byways of research are sometimes laughable, often immodest. I experimented with toilet seats, tipping them down in back. By placing several thicknesses of foam rubber between the front of the toilet seat and the bowl, the seat tipped up in front and caused the "sitter" to come close to the squat position as he voided his bowels.

In one house that I built I met the disapproving looks of the builder, and especially the "master plumber" when I insisted on setting the bowl of the toilet in concrete at a severe down-tipped angle. Had I gone loco? I could see the wonder in their eyes. The entire project was a nuisance, I admit. Our whole society is built on the premise that furnishings must look nice, no matter if they cause discomfort and even disease.

PUTTING IT ALL TOGETHER

If you have any worry that your bowel evacuations are not complete, try in some way to have your BMs in a squat-like position. Do not artificially wash out your bowels with enemas, high colonics or such. These tend to disturb the fluid balance of the body. They also tend to push out the lower rectum into a retaining sac for uneliminated waste material and create double trouble for constipated people. If pregnant, lean acutely forward while seated at stool. This will allow the womb to shift forward so that it does not kink or dent the rectal tube.

Chapter Six

Blood Transfusions

The reader may be startled to learn that blood transfusions are not universally considered to be desirable. They may not even be especially scientific.

If you have ever had a blood transfusion, or given a pint of blood, you deserve to know some things that you never hear about. There are vastly differing opinions and views about the matter. The following, for example.

The life is in the blood; therefore whatever diseases or tendencies a person has are also resident in his blood.

If a tendency toward drunkenness is in the blood, then whoever receives a transfusion of such a chronic alcoholic's blood will also inherit the tendency toward alcoholism. So goes the scientific opinion in some quarters—one the lay person never hears at all.

Whether a person has a tendency toward kleptomania, a genetic leaning toward skin rashes, a diathesis toward nervous tension or a fear of heights, all this is held to be ingrained in the blood pattern. This being so—and it sounds trustworthily right as rain—just consider the innocent one who receives within his bloodstream an admixture from such a donor. Does not the donor's blood then transfer such unhappy characteristics and tendencies to the recipient of his blood?

You see, don't you, that there is a side to the business of blood transfusions that is very hush-hush. But in an area that may affect our future life and all our future generations we deserve to know all the facts.

If this subject interests you, you will want to read the following pages and perhaps light a candle for others by giving a little informative speech on the subject to your favorite organization or service club.

***

Startling Research in Blood Transfusions

The lay person who hears about the four major blood groupings known as blood types, and even more about the Rh-positive (and Rh-negative) individuals than about the A, B, O and AB groups themselves, has no idea how wide of the actual mark this entire blood-grouping business falls.

The fact is that there are as many blood types as there are people. In gross and very general groupings there may be only four blood types, yes. But please consider that your own blood chemistry is not exactly compatible with any other person's on earth. Not even with the blood chemistry of your own children. You are *you,* unblendingly *you,* with a blood chemistry as individually your own as your fingerprints. No one else on this planet has the blood characteristics peculiar to the blood that flows in your arteries and veins.

The life is in the blood. That's the way the Bible says it and that's the way it is. Your characteristics, good and bad, and all your genetic inheritances, are there in the blood.

When you donate blood, the recipient receives from you the tendencies and inheritances that have made you *you.* Do you have, or have you ever had, a tubercular diathesis? Are you the victim of any allergies? Does it "run in your family" as a kind of family trait to have rheumatic miseries, or are all of you as a family given to developing heart trouble if you develop any trouble at all? What do you suppose happens with all these genetic and personal strains in your blood when you donate a pint of it? Does the recipient have a strainer in his metabolic factory to filter them out?

This book is written in popular language rhythms but it is a scientific book, so let us boldly come to grips with the scientific realities. Ready? Then be assured of this.

When you undergo a blood transfusion you receive the donor's tendencies toward drunkenness, toward kleptomania, toward skin rashes or visual defects or a fear of heights or whatever.

It has been correctly said that originality is merely a pair of fresh eyes. All this that I am writing about here would better be left unsaid if there were nothing else we could do about it—no other technique available to us. If that's the best we can do, that's it. When we are dying from lack of blood let us be thankful that there are blood banks to save our lives, even if there's a possibility of inheriting bad things along with the life-saving ones.

But there is another way. A smarter way. A way that offers incalculable rewards by way of eliminating the chance of another's unwanted blood factors becoming our own. Let us take a look with fresh eyes.

Some years ago I communicated with a renowned surgeon who had a 125-bed hospital near Boston. In 43 years this man had performed over 20,000 surgeries, doing the surgical work for some 400 allopathic doctors, mostly from Boston, who were not themselves surgeons. This man was Dr. Alonzo J. Shadman, a medical man of great stature.

The Surgeon Who Refuses to Use Blood Transfusions

Dr. Shadman had read a book of mine and wrote me a con-gratulatory note. He said he'd like me to help him put together a book of his own, and we corresponded. In one of his letters he set forth the startling ideas of not using blood transfusions in surgery, and his reasons therefor. I share them with you here.

Human life began in the sea. Human blood is salted to the degree of normal saline solution. Since taking on a load of anyone else's blood is at best dangerous—for there is no such thing as absolute blood compatibility but only relative accom-modative compatibility—why not use transfusions of normal saline to start up the body's own blood-making apparatus so that the body manufactures its own (compatible) type of blood?

In his own practice Dr. Shadman had given up ordinary blood transfusions some 15 years earlier, using only normal saline transfusions instead. And with what results? Hear the words of the surgeon himself.

"Since going exclusively to normal saline transfusions," he wrote to me, "I have never lost a case because of blood-lack. Even accident cases that were brought into the surgery in exsanguinated states [chalk-white from loss of blood] never died from such lack of blood."

Significant? The man's surgery schedule was heavy. No blood transfusions were employed. Yet not a single case did he lose from changing over to saline water transfusions.

PUTTING IT ALL TOGETHER

The advice is simple—and obvious. If a blood transfusion becomes your lot, and you just cannot convince the ruling doctor-in-chief to do it any other way, be sure to get blood from a known source. I would rule out a blood bank. I would not want blood from just anyone. The safest measure in the circumstances is to solicit a blood donation from a person you know, and whose living habits you are acquainted with, and whose personality—especially this!—you like.

Chapter Seven

The Question of the Cold Plunge

Many persons are plagued with arthritic pains, or lingering coughs or other miseries, persons who had been great athletes in their youth.

They cannot understand it.

"How can it be?" they ask. "In college I was a track star (or football giant) and laid in enough good health during those formative years to last me, wouldn't you say?"

Are you one of those, and do you think like that?

The answer is that you do not and cannot "lay in" a stock of health for the future, for one year of indiscretions can wash away three previous decades of good behavior. But one thing needs to be known. In youth you have the vigor and resistance to take punishment and bounce back into relative health. All those football jarrings and pummelings may not have seemed to affect you then—but they did in fact take their toll. Now, in middle age, you feel the strains and stresses that your organism was punished with in youthful days.

Perhaps you can do next to nothing now about what happened in the long ago. That may be true. But do you have children? Or grandchildren? And would not your present mellow wisdom be useful in guiding them *away* from bodily shocks and neurological "unwisdoms" that they cannot see or gauge with youthful eyes?

Sound sensible? Read on.

***

Researching the Cold Plunge

I had a patient who in his youth had been what he called a Polar Bear. This means he'd gone out in the dead of winter and cavorted in the ocean with his fellow polar bears. Actually in snowy and icy weather, wearing only bathing trunks, actually plunging into the frigid ocean several mornings a week.

Now he was in middle age and wanted to know if his daily ice-cold shower was a good practice to continue. But I was treating him for a trifacial neuralgia and he had other signs of having overpunished his nervous system.

"Would you permit me to lecture you a bit?" I asked the man. He knew by my tone that I was in no mood to approve his heroic activities. "Cold showers and cold plunges are not advisable," I told him. "They are shocks to the nervous system."

He told me again that he hardly ever had a cold because of the daily cold bath. I saw he was trying to justify his youthful pranks. It was necessary to set him straight—get him to share a research project I'd already completed.

What follows is what I told the man.

My entire approach to human physiology, and especially neurology, is at its finest and best in my willingness to *listen to the wisdom of the body*. When the body tells you that you're sleepy, go to bed and do not defer it until you have finished that hand at bridge or read that final chapter. If your body signals a desire to urinate, don't wait until you have written that letter or finished the long telephone conversation.

Think of yourself on the beach even on a very hot day. Note how you react instinctively when, to test the temperature of the water, you experimentally dip one toe into the sea. You draw back by instinct. Your entire body rejects the cold. The nerve impulses rush to your brain and say *Don't!* That's your innate intelligence (your neurological wisdom) at work.

But then your "educated intelligence" takes over. It reminds you that after an icy plunge into the sea you'll experience a quick reaction of glowing warmth. Your skin and whole body will tingle. So you ignore "the wisdom of the body" and plunge in.

What happened when your body reacted with a tingling sense of warmth and euphoria was a body defense mechanism to protect itself from harm. It was a neurologically directed self-preservation reaction to protect the organism against an inimical environment. The nervous system ordered all the pores to close tight. Bodily heat was retained. The internal furnace adapted to your "educated foolishness" until balance of the thermogenic centers could be restored.

Human life, it appears, began in the tropics. The organism thrives best in warmth, must strenuously accommodate itself to cold. Thrusting yourself into a cold pool will bring a sense of glowing warmth as a defensive reaction—but this happens only in youth and in reasonably good health, when the reserve stores are sufficient to take such shocks. In poor health it is devitalizing and dangerous. In all cases it is a neurological shock to throw your warm body into very cold water.

PUTTING IT ALL TOGETHER

The very best temperature for a bath is that which is most nearly like the 98.6° of the human body. When the water surrounding you is within a degree or two of the temperature inside the body itself, the body is at ease. The opposite to ease is *dis*-ease. Disease, meaning lack of bodily ease, makes for functional distress, uses up restorative powers. Bodily wisdom rules out cold plunges.

Chapter Eight

A Discovery in
Breast Self-Examination

Everywhere, in every female group, the subject of mastectomies comes up. Mastectomies are surgical operations.

It's hard to believe that at times lumps in the female breast can be taken care of naturally and effectively.

If you are a female reader, you have had plenty of reason lately to become frightened of cancer of the breast. The papers and networks mention the subject daily. You are urged to have your breasts examined for lumps in the mammary tissue right now, without loss of time, *pronto*.

But—hold on a minute. Suppose you knew of a perfectly natural, and sensible, and *physiologically correct* way to take care of this. Such a way exists. It takes only a week or two to try out the method—and if it works, as it certainly does so very beautifully and so often—look at the anguish and expense and scarring surgery that is saved.

In the following few pages the method is spelled out in earnest. If you are a woman, or if you have women friends or even growing female children, you will want to know about this research adventure in the field of lumps in the breast.

***

An Adventure in the Field of Lumps in the Breast

I am sure that now is the time to finally publish my own research findings in the area of breast lumps.

It had to do with my purchasing a room full of cold white lights. These variously shaped lights were used to inspect and examine the sinuses, mastoids, even teeth at the gumline and below the gumline to detect abscesses and other trouble in the making. The patient was placed in a completely dark room—an annex to the dark room of my X-ray developing room, in fact—and when the strong white light contacted the suspected area there ensued such intense transillumination as to make one gasp. The interior tissues showed up with unexpectedly meaningful signs of health or lack of health, as the case might be. The large investment in the transillumination room of my clinic became a subject of conversation among doctors.

Then, by sheer chance, I began using the white lights to transilluminate female breasts. Sitting in the dark room and facing a wall mirror, the patient could not only see her own network of vessels in the mammary gland while I was examining it, but if lumps were present she could also see opaque white patches easily recognizable to her as different, in an ugly way, from the pink flesh tones of the healthy tissues.

In those days it did not really matter to me whether the lumps would test out as malignant or benign. Since the very act of doing the biopsy has been known to trigger cancer all by itself, I wished to avoid biopsies wherever possible. But I knew one thing, then another sure thing, then a third dependable thing.

One, the lumpy mass in the breast was a collection of protein; protein *accumulated*, and *uneliminated,* in the mammary gland. Two, if I disallowed the eating of protein for a week or so, then the body itself would tend to "eat up" the stored protein masses residing in its interior. Three, since my other researches in short fasting schedules and mono-diet programs proved to my satisfaction that fasting or mono-dieting for a single week would harm no one, I might have stumbled onto a research find of enormous value.

Use a Flashlight to Illuminate Breasts

This project led to the use of ordinary flashlights in place of my expensive white-light, cold-light equipment. A mother asked how she could get her daughter in a distant state to see her own breasts as she, the mother, has seen them in my dark room. Experimentally, a strong flashlight was suggested. It worked. All that was needed was a fairly dark closet in which to examine oneself. It was later found that almost any closet could have the chinks of light plugged and made to serve.

Most important, it seemed to me, was to get rid of the fright element. I hammered at patients with this saying: *"Worrying in advance of an event is like paying interest on a note before it falls due."* I showed them the books of the illustrations of Dr. Crile of the Cleveland Neurological Clinic which declares that those breast lump cases that undergo operations and those that don't live just about equally as long. In these days, with this widespread breast cancer panic, I wish above all to eliminate the fear and terror from women's minds.

PUTTING IT ALL TOGETHER

First, obtain a strong flashlight with a lens sufficiently wide to let the underpart of your breast rest upon it. Then close yourself into a dark, very dark closet, and place the light under your breast. Looking down upon the entire breast you'll see a network of vessels (veins, etc.) that may frighten you, but they are perfectly healthy and natural. Very rarely you may see a lump or milky mass among the clear breast tissue. They may be only temporary mammary congestions that leave as automatically as they formed. But they can also be serious—so then what?

Take a week away from consuming protein-rich foods. Compel your body to consume its own store of resident proteins, such as the protein mass in the breast. Eliminate meat, fish, eggs, cheese, nuts, milk. If you have the discipline for it, the best single experiment is to fast for a week, taking nothing but water, preferably distilled water, and that only in small amounts, just enough to quench thirst. If you cannot undergo fasting, eat only as large a variety of fruits for a week as you desire—nothing but fruits, and preferably all you want of only *one* fruit at a meal—21 different fruits in the week if you like.

At the end of a week go into that dark closet and have another look. With no proteins having been consumed, more often than not, you will find that the body ate up its own stored protein and the breast is now clear. Pink and healthy all throughout! Try it for a week. Time enough to do biopsies and suchlike later if this doesn't work.

Chapter Nine

Chewing and Digestion

Are you worried about indigestion and bad breath?

Are you generally a cranky individual?

Are you a gum-chewer—what some people have come to label a "gum-aholic"?

And do you have a sour feeling in the stomach, as though a fermenting factory were alive down in that region?

All of the foregoing may quite possibly be related and interrelated beyond anything you have ever dreamed. Of course, you would not be expected to know this. The sweet-talking ads tell you that gum-chewing—especially chewing their brand of gum—refreshes the breath. "It aids digestion" is what the ads also (and nervily!) claim.

Not being a physiologist, how would you as a layman know that the very act of chewing gum may be *causing* your indigestion, and also your bad breath?

Yet this is in many instances the actual case, and here follows an explanation that you will probably never forget.

***

Research Adventure: How People Chew Gum into Sickness

Some patients smoke and cannot stop. Others chew gum and have made a habit of it. This thirty-ish lady came into the office chewing madly on her gum, and when leaving the first thing she did was open the pack and extract a fresh stick of gum.

Suddenly the impact of her health-destroying habit hit me hard. She was manufacturing her own indigestion! No wonder she complained of bad breath, frequent constipation, dependence on laxatives. The very gum which she chomped all day to sweeten the breath was making her breath foul and contributing to her constipation.

Here was a little-known cause for poor digestion. People who chewed gum swallowed saliva constantly. Saliva contains a starch digesting enzyme (ptyalin) manufactured in the salivary glands. By swallowing a steady flow of ptyalin-containing saliva the gum chewers overwork the manufacturing glands. Then, when they eat starchy foods like wheat, corn, potatoes and the like there isn't enough of the enzyme around to digest these things completely. By chewing gum all day long they've *fooled* the system into manufacturing this starch-digesting enzyme for no good reason at all.

Chewing gum, be it said loud and clear, does not aid digestion as the advertising has it. The exact opposite is true. Now hat this simple but important truth is set forth, I hope the reader will not be a reservoir *but a pipeline,* and share it with friends and loved ones.

The lady whose gum chewing had started this adventure in research was of Scottish ancestry and accustomed to having her porridge every morning. Others who ate oatmeal or other starch cereals were also addicted to the purportedly "refreshing" gum chewing habit. And quite often their complaint in the clinic was of a digestive nature.

When they were put under strict instructions to abandon the habit, their digestion in most cases improved and their breath actually became sweeter. This was because the starchy items in their food were now properly prepared for stomach digestion through a sufficiency of ptyalin in the mouth. No longer were they stimulating the manufacture of this starch enzyme and swallowing it with no digestive purpose whatever.

A side result of this was a sweeter disposition among cranky patients with digestive complaints. Heretofore their starchy foods were not properly prepared for stomach digestion, so the foods fermented and soured in the stomach. This made for sour dispositions besides poor plumbing setups. When the chewing of gum was halted, however, we proved that many conditions are somatico-psychic rather than psychosomatic; that is, the body was influencing the mind and emotions rather than the other way around.

PUTTING IT ALL TOGETHER

You must first of all be aware that Step One in starch digestion takes place in the mouth, and that the enzyme for this is in the saliva. Therefore, saliva should not be swallowed for hours on end, as happens when we chew gum. Save the saliva for the times when starchy food items are eaten: breads, potatoes, bananas, corn, cereals, all grains and flour products. When you quit gum chewing, do not go to a substitute habit, as some have done. People who were addicted to gum and ordered to stop sometimes took up sucking on a peach pit or similar object. They continued to swallow saliva needlessly and harmfully. Besides, this was often oral tension and better foregone. Hearkening back to the mother's breast is not for adults.

Chapter Ten

Danger in the Bathroom

Are you one of those persons who always seems to have his or her eyes infected and reinfected? And, besides, do you have weakish gums that somehow feel tainted?

Well, would you believe that your bathroom is not correctly designed? After all these years and authentically great architectural advances, yes—they still don't know how to design a bathroom that accords with human health needs. Toothbrushes are given little holes to hang in, but in the wrong place. They should hang inside a medicine cabinet, not outside where the toothbrush bristles can absorb all the bacteria that "perfumes" bathrooms with such powerful odors so very frequently.

***

Remarkable Research Find: Where to Hang Toothbrushes

This adventure in research came about in a curious way. The lady asked why it was that her husband left such a strong odor behind him in the bathroom after an evacuation of the bowel. In the same bit of dialogue she mentioned how she came to observe this.

"I have a hang-up about brushing my teeth," she said. It was almost an apology. "I guess I run into the bathroom a dozen times a day to scrub my teeth—after every mouthful I consume—and I notice this foul smell hanging on after Charles has his bowel movements."

A long time before I had learned some valuable lessons about how to treat sick people. One was this: Treat the patient, not the condition. Another was this: Listen well to what patients have to tell you; often you learn more from them than they do from you.

What the lady had said caught in my head and nibbled at my brain. Why was there a noticeably foul odor after her husband's stool? The most reasonable cause for it must be an over-consumption of protein foods. I must ask if he eats a lot of eggs, cheese, fish and meat every day, drinking some of it down with more protein in the form of milk. If so, I'll just have to explain that whatever protein one uses that's beyond the body's daily limit of some sixty grams to utilize, all such surplus protein must undergo putrefaction. When it putrefies it forms those three stinky acids: indol, skatol and phenol (carbolic) acid.

Suddenly the entire matter clicked. It became important. The odors of the three acids persisted in the room because the foul bacteria lingered in the air and could be smelled by those who entered. This woman entered the bathroom to brush her teeth. Her toothbrush hung conveniently exposed outside the medicine cabinet where she could reach it. Didn't those foul bacteria also crawl inside the bristles of her toothbrush?

Didn't she unknowingly dig befouled bristles into her teeth and gum margins as she brushed so assiduously?

And her towels, did they not also hang where they were handy to grab? Hanging outside any cabinet, did they not also absorb the smelly bacteria in the room?

People rub their eyes with such free-hanging towels that may be absorbing unwanted bacterial life. People ought to be warned about it. This has never been researched. It could not be classed as any earth-shaking piece of research, but people of delicacy and refinement would appreciate this bit of information.

PUTTING IT ALL TOGETHER

The way we plan our bathrooms needs a re-examination and a serious rethink. In Chapter Five I told how I had found that the backs of toilet seats ought to be tipped downward. Now I find that medicine cabinets ought to be much larger than they are. Bathroom closets should be built to contain all towels and toothbrushes.

Any exposed item in the bathroom that you apply to the face or skin or eyes ought to be closeted in an air-tight locker or closet. Nothing that is employed in intimate use should ever hang exposed. Besides this, of course, all lingering foul odors after bowel evacuations ought to be run down to cause. Are they due to a serious bowel or rectal condition? Are they due to overeating protein foods?

Usually it is the latter.

Chapter Eleven

A Simple Aid for Arteriosclerosis
and the Elderly

The elderly patient who had his wife doing all the talking for him showed signs of arteriosclerosis, or hardening of the arteries.

He was very slow in his responses, somewhat hesitant in his answers, often forgetful of what he had started to say. Most of the time he sat beside his wife with a blank expression, as though absent from the scene.

"I do everything for his comfort that I know how to do," she explained. "His room is light and bright and clean. The bed is comfortable. The pillows are fluffed out and high to support his back, the way he likes them and the way they showed me in the spa in Europe."

The woman's chance remark about the pillows piled high for her husband's back started a chain of thought processes. Indeed, it triggered a small research project. She had taken her husband to an expensive sanitarium in Switzerland and had been shown, among other things, how to get him comfortable, raised quite high on a pile of pillows. This was the custom in many otherwise efficient hospitals and spas in Europe, as it was here at home also.

But it was wrong. It was harmful to the patient with hardening of the arteries. It was *physiologically* as unsuitable to his needs as could be!

The first thing I instructed the man to do was to *lower* his head from time to time during the day. "Do most of your resting on a level surface," I counseled. "Forget about being boosted up on pillows. Your brain only works when it is given oxygen. And the oxygen comes to it from the blood. And the blood doesn't reach the brain easily when the head is way up high."

They nodded with understanding. The wife caught it at once, the husband a bit more slowly.

"Here is my advice," I continued. "Refresh your brain cells and your arteries with more oxygen from time to time by lying crosswise on the bed, face down, with the head hanging over the edge of the bed *lower* than the body. Think of yourself as looking for shoes under the bed. Do this five minutes at a time say three or four times a day." What I was saying appeared easy to grasp for again they nodded with enthusiasm. "I will give you other instructions later, but for now get into the habit of resting your body on the level, and occasionally with the head lower, not high on pillows."

It was laughably simple advice. But on their next visit they reported a little progress. Of added benefit was something we hadn't counted on: The elderly gentleman took an interest in this. To him it was a game; he actually looked forward to something at last—even if it was merely a session of lying face down on the bed with his head lowered.

The arteriosclerotic man was told to do other things to help nourish his slow-acting brain. "For additional value," I urged, "give yourself a physiological treat by resting on the carpet on the floor a few times a day on your knees and elbows. Lower your head. Bring the chest down to where it is below the level of your hips. While in this position try to part your lips and pant like a dog."

I explained that this will exercise the diaphragm and tend to strengthen the entire breathing apparatus. I also advised the daily consumption of lecithin and wheat germ as a cereal dish with skimmed milk, for in wheat germ and lecithin existed all the ingredients needed by human brain cells. And he was ordered to take long daily walks, walking slowly if need be at first, and to count twice as long exhaling as inhaling. This seemed difficult to get across to them.

"Get into the habit of counting to yourself as you walk," I said. "When you take the breath in count to four or five, let us say. When letting out the breath be sure to count at the same speed to eight or ten. Thus your exhalations will take double the time of your inhalations. This tightens the breathing muscles and strengthens them. It will teach your body to oxygenate better."

The man tried it right there in the office and his eyes glistened. It was fun; it was useful; it was absolutely consistent with his physiological needs.

PUTTING IT ALL TOGETHER

It is a specious argument that elderly people need the most rest and therefore merit the best, fattest pillows to rest upon. But human blood flows best on a level plane. Those who suffer from arteriosclerosis already are short of oxygen in the brain. The oxygen they need can reach them only through the blood. A better, easier blood-flow therefore is desirable and unquestionably scientific. Thus it follows that people with hardened arteries, which already have a smaller than normal carrying capacity, should not boost up their heads on large pillows. They should rest on a level surface where the blood and brain-nourishing oxygen can reach the cranial areas without difficulty. When I asked patients with arteriosclerosis to get into positions where the blood-flow was made easier to the cranial organs, most of them felt perkier, quicker and more mentally alert very rapidly. If you have memory lapses at times, even if you are not yet old (for nowadays we note hardened arteries even in youngish persons), it cannot hurt to give the above mentioned drills a try. Hang your head *down* over the side of a bed. Get into the restful position on your knees and elbows. Do diaphragmatic breathing. Count twice as long exhaling as inhaling.

And please do not fail to note this: If you take as little as one teaspoonful of wheat germ oil daily it is almost equivalent to getting under an oxygen tent, as discovered recently by some researchers.

And by all means try to avoid the "simple" sugars such as molasses, honey, cane sugar, syrups. During the time of your self-treatment, it you wish to live up to this book's title and reach pain-free health and longevity, confine yourself to the complex sugars such as dried beans, wheat germ, grains such as brown rice, whole barley, whole rye.

And male readers with prostate difficulties, take note of this most especially: For your protein needs take mostly pumpkin seeds. Buy them hulled and eat them that way or, if you have a chewing problem, grind them into a powdery consistency in a blender or grinder. Why pumpkin seeds? Because some studies among gypsy tribes in southern Europe revealed that there was no identifiable prostate gland trouble among its men—and this was traced to their habit of eating pumpkin seeds all day long just as some of us here chew peanuts throughout the day.

One final instruction. It would generally be helpful to take about 200 International Units of vitamin E after meals. Take this after the oiliest meal of the day if you take it only once a day—after the meal with a salad that has oily salad dressing in it, for example. And when you consume vitamin E do not take any iron tablets, for it appears that they cancel each other out. Therefore, if you take blackstrap molasses, for instance, because of its rich, utilizable iron content, take this at bedtime when it does not interfere with your vitamin E consumption.

Chapter Twelve

Avoiding Dyspepsia and the Dowager's Hump

Are you affected with dyspepsia or indigestion? A victim of stomach distress? Deficient in hydrochloric acid?

Do you eat every meal half afraid of the suffering you will have later for the joy of eating that you experience now?

Well, just listen to this. There is good news for you in two well-defined areas. Now we know how to instruct you in a single and simple little exercise that will beat the world as a digestive aid. It will straighten your spine, and thereby unpinch the pressure you probably have on nerves that lead to your stomach or other digestive organs. With a free, unhampered flow of nerve impulses to digestive organs, they'll receive the "juice" for their work and then tend to function normally. That's No. 1.

No. 2 is something else which is very simple, remarkably effective in almost every case, and requires only two weeks to accomplish. The first week is spent in fasting. This will give your damaged areas of the digestive apparatus a perfect physiological rest, and a chance to get self-repaired. The second week is spent on a diet of only fruits.

It is a fascinating program. And as a bonus you will get acquainted with the "Dowager's Hump" on the following two or three pages.

***

An Unsettling Research Adventure into Dyspepsia and the Dowager's Hump

They were a loving, hand-holding couple of middle age. The lady was stout, pale, and had eyes with concern in them. The man was cadaverously skinny, round-shouldered in a way that emphasized his sunken chest, but he was a jaunty and humor-loving gentleman just the same.

"I'm a long-time HCl-man," he told me with a kind of curious pride, for he had taken enough hydrochloric acid for his stomach problems to know how to discuss it chemically.

The man did not show signs of achlorhydria, which is an entire absence of hydrochloric acid in the stomach and can betoken a serious anemia (pernicious). Thus, the function was alive, only it was not alive enough. His stoop indicated the strong possibility of pressure in the mid-spine on nerves that energized the stomach. If this actually existed in his vertebral column, then the gastric glands in his stomach were not receiving enough nerve power through the pinched nerves to manufacture the needed hydrochloric acid—an acid that serves a variety of functions in the digestive process.

An Easy Way to Align Your Spine

It was an easy matter to run down. I'd soon find out.

"You have what I call a Dowager's Hump," I told him. "I will advise an exercise that will move every vertebra in the middle of your spine inward, forward, out of that rounded slouch you've got."

I asked him to clasp his hands behind his back, palms touching, then roll his elbows inward until they nearly touched. He touched the elbows behind his back and immediately the chest came up as the spine straightened. On being instructed to keep rolling and unrolling his elbows, bringing them inward and outward, the man became enthusiastic. He peeked into the mirror and was gladdened by the look of his chest as it came up out of its dished-in hollow, and of his spine as it came up in a kind of military bearing.

There is hardly any point in extending the story here. The matter did prove to be what I'd observed in other similar digestive syndromes: pinched nerves causing a digestive incapacity. In this case it was a lack of hydrochloric acid; in others the nerve pressures manifested themselves in a large variety of digestive upsets and stomach distresses.

I asked the man also to give his metabolic factory a good rest by going on only fruits for a week, eating the way primates eat in their natural state. He did so. He also did the Dowager's Hump drill with frequency and enthusiasm. He stopped taking his dilute hydrochloric acid tablets. No longer was he "an HCl man."

PUTTING IT ALL TOGETHER

Drugs for digestive troubles constitute a road without any ending. The digestive processes are always, without exception, directed by nerve impulses, and the nerve pathways which transfer such impulses can be pinched or blocked at the spine. In cases of stoop shoulders this is very evident. But spinal nerve pressures may exist on the nerve pathways to the stomach even in those with ramrod-straight vertebral columns. It cannot possibly hurt, and may do all the good you seek, to go through the drill that I've called The Dowager's Hump Exercise. Just clasp your hands together in back with palms touching and roll the elbows inward with vigor. Do this several times daily. Do 15 to 20 of these rolls at bedtime.

In addition, for nearly every digestive problem, a one-week fast is useful. It gives the body a beneficial physiological rest. While fasting, do not be very active *in any way*. Take a week out of your life to do nothing at all: no reading, writing letters, listening to radios, any of the things that use up a measure of energy. Save all that energy for the purpose at hand, by which I mean repairing the damaged cells and tissues. Just lie in a dark or semidark room for a week and let the body repair itself. After that, try a week only on fruits. By thus unpinching the accumulated nerve pressures and also normalizing the digestive capacity you will be more likely to attain digestive health than by anything else ever discovered in my 40 years of doctoring.

Chapter Thirteen

The Harmfulness of
One-Sided Exercise

The following pages are for those who suffer, or have ever suffered, the pangs and pains of sciatica. They are also for people with the kind of low back problem that is commonly called sacroiliac trouble. Besides this, what follows is of special benefit to those who have leg pains on the outer portion of the thigh going clear down to the arch of the foot.

If readers with the aforementioned ailments will read, *and heed,* they may quickly discover that this book bears a quite correct title. With rare exceptions the well-planned and carefully researched methods of relief and benefits will in fact prove to be, as the title indicates, *a miracle guide to pain-free health and longevity.*

The pain of sciatica can be so intense that it really shortens life, thus affecting longevity. The sciatic nerve (along with the vagus nerve) is just about the longest in the body and certainly the thickest and fattest—meaning that pain in this nerve pathway can mean a great deal of pain. On the very same day three men came into my office with the three excruciatingly painful ailments I just mentioned. And each one was helped in the manner I am about to describe.

The middle-aged sciatica sufferer was quite athletic and an enthusiastic golfer. His misery was almost unbearable. I discovered that in this man, as in many sciatica cases, the giant sciatic nerve was being pressed upon, and also rubbed, by the hard bony rim of what is called the sciatic notch.

Real suffering there. It meant that the body's softest tissue, *nerve tissue,* suffered the friction and insult of being rubbed by the hardest tissue in the human body, *bone tissue.* This man's sciatic nerve, instead of being in the middle of the sciatic notch of the pelvis, where it would be unmolested, had swung or been worked to the side where it rubbed against the actual bony rim and suffered raw pain. I knew what to do.

Stretch the Sciatic Nerve Away from the Wrong Position

I ordered the man to lie flat on his back on the floor, facing the wall, then raise his hurting leg and rest the heel of that leg against the wall. To do this I asked him to take a position close to the wall, facing it squarely, and then to raise the painful leg with the knee stiff; that is, the leg locked and straight instead of bent. As the man did this I urged him to wiggle his body closer to the wall so that the leg was closer and closer to the wall. As he worked his buttocks nearest to the wall the sciatica-ridden leg came higher up on the wall, stretching the sciatic nerve. After a few minutes in this position the nerve was apparently worked back into the center of the notch, away from contact with the bony rim of the notch, and the man's pain-etched face relaxed.

He smiled at me wanly and the first thing he said was that perhaps now, at long last, he again could get in a round of golf.

Something inside me clicked. Since I am by impluse and discipline a researcher, his remark caused me to ask myself a pertinent question: *What relationship could there be between his golfing and his sciatica?* I showed him how to get down on his hands and knees and force the lower back to sway down as low as possible, then arch repeatedly upward as high as possible, thus unpinching the pinched nerves in the lower spine, then went about my work with other patients. But the thought about golfing—which is really a one-sided sport because the force of the swing is usually on one side of the pelvis—kept nibbling and gnawing on the periphery of my mind.

The Technique for Sacroiliac Sufferers

Leaving our golfing enthusiast, I went into the room occupied by a religiously avid bowling league man, another middle-ager with lancinating pains in his right sacroiliac joint. He could hardly move a step. Even the act of taking a breath caused a knife-like pain to stab him in the sacroiliac articulation.

I instructed the poor man to get down on hands and knees, as in the case of the golfer. But here, instead of ordering him to sway and arch the lower back, I ordered him to keep lifting the left side of his pelvis with vigor. As he energetically boosted up the side of his hip opposite to where the pain was, the articulating spines of the sacroiliac joint found their correct juxtaposition and the severe nerve-pressure-pain subsided. Then I advised the man to quit being a right-handed bowler for a time and actually bowl with his left hand. This reversed the strains and balanced up both sacroiliac articulations. Following this, I said, he could play his serious bowling league games with his mighty right arm, but afterward, when each game was finished, he just had to play a round or two with his left arm to keep the pelvic parts balanced.

As I left the sacroiliac case for the next patient my mind dwelled again on the factor of one-sidedness. The researcher in me was alerted. H'mmm. The sciatica case was a golf enthusiast who swung backward to *some degree,* but then forward to a *terrific degree*—always straining in this one way, always forcing the sciatic nerve away from the center of the notch toward the bony hard rim. Finally the man's sciatic nerve touched the rim of the notch, rubbed against it with every movement, became raw and pain-filled from the friction and pressure. No wonder. The man just had to be instructed to learn occasional swings in the other directions, with the strains *reversed.*

The bowling man with very severe sacroiliac pain did powerful lunges forward with his *right hand* and hurled the heavy ball down the alley against the *right pelvic articulations.* The germinal idea began to cook. Things were adding up.

I entered the room where the dentist nursed his toothache-like syndrome. On the outer side of his left thigh (vastus lateralis) he had this grinding, unceasing low-grade pain. This man also was middle-aged. He had two strikes against him: one, he was an active tennis player; two, he worked sideways, as all dentists do, forever leaning in one direction over his patients' mouths. Of the several hundred dentists that I have treated in a long career there was never one I could recall who did not have trouble in the mid- to upper-thoracic spinal column. Some had what we call an incipient lateral scoliosis, which is a kind of vertebral curvature. This patient had a well-defined curvature that is characteristic of those who habitually do their jobs leaning in a single direction. They also, I have observed, often have stomach trouble and vague digestive ills; and this, I am sure, is traceable to the fact that the nerve pathways to the digestive organs emerge from the spinal cord between vertebrae in this area to feed the organs with nerve impulses. Without these nerve impulses nothing happens. They are the "juice" for the motor; they provide both the functional power and the directions that guide digestive organs in their work.

I studied the dentist a moment. Beads of sweat from the pain were on his upper lip. As he spoke with soft lovingness about his tennis he probably never considered that the one-sidedness of the movement and the strains of serving the tennis ball, driving that ball over the net with enormous vigor, could be connected with his leg pain, just as the occupational one-sidedness of his work at the dental chair daily contributed to the leg syndrome, as well as to the upper spinal curvature that was already forming.

Tennis . . . and Digestive Problems . . . and Leg Pains

The connection between one-sided tennis and leg pains and digestive ills kept burrowing into my mind as I observed the dentist nursing his slow, grinding, unstoppable pain. Later it was he who called it "a toothache in the entire leg." He kept rubbing the side of his thigh and clenching his jaw from the pain, that unceasing, low-grade but maddening ache.

This man was also middle aged. (Funny about the middle years: With the vigor of youth you could stand the wallops of football and the neurological shocks of cold plunges and the strains of one-sided sports with no apparent harm. You had the resistance to bounce back. But when I saw them in my office in later years I could see the jarring impacts and strains and stresses of earlier years showing up. They showed up in *structural faults* of the body. This was my special area of competence. This I had unfailingly observed.)

The dentist burped and placed his hand on his stomach. He mentioned faulty digestion and another hook-up thought came to me. I remembered that many tennis players who'd come to the office also complained of digestive problems. Could it be because they served the ball one-sidedly, twisting the spine always in one direction, thereby pinching nerves there that lead out between vertebrae to the digestive organs?

As I indicated, our dental doctor had two strikes against him: As an active tennis player he forever pushed his body with great vigor from one side only to the opposite side as he served his tennis balls; as a dentist he forever leaned in one direction over his patients. It was necessary to order him to cease forthwith all efforts in his beloved game. At this he made a wry face and shook his head.

On explaining precisely why I ordered this (for in doctoring I'd learned that explanations get the best patient participation and cooperation, especially when the instructions are unusual), he complied with reluctance. I did urge upon him, however, to lob the ball over the net *with his left hand,* just for the sake of practice and some exposure to sun and air. Then he was told to lie flat on his back and swing the stiff right leg across the body at about the groin area, and to do this repeatedly until somewhat tired. Especially at bedtime was it necessary to do this, for what one gains at bedtime one tends to retain during bedtime, when bodily injuries and strains are repaired.

Technique for the Internal Chemistry

In all these cases it is also necessary to take care of the "internal plumbing" as well as re-establish the structural alignment that takes pressures off nerves and puts joints back where they belong.

The dentist had digestive problems. The bowling man and the golfer had, in common with the dentist, plenty of nerve pain, irritated and screaming nerve ends. They needed a program that would make their internal environment free of irritants and toxins. When this was done along with correcting the structural faults of their bodies they could hardly help but get well.

First off, therefore, all cases of *sciatica* and *sacroiliac* trouble and *leg pain*—all were ordered to stop the use of spices, especially no pepper, mustard, chilis, any bitey foods.

They were forbidden the use of carbonated drinks, all kinds of very cold drinks or foods, nothing for a short time (until they got well) that was much colder than room temperature. They were positively prohibited from taking alcohol in any form, not even "a little wine for their stomach's sake."

A pair of Texas researchers had discovered great value in cherries for gout, but I'd found that a meal of just a half pound of cherries, preferably for breakfast as the sole food, aided in almost all cases where there was great pain being suffered. I instructed these three middle-agers to eat a half pound or more of either fresh ripe cherries or even canned Bing cherries for breakfast—and nothing else.

I had long before this discovered that high protein diets prolong the agony of painful maladies—and also discovered why. The body is severely limited to being able to metabolize or utilize some 50 grams of protein daily, and any amount over that almost always undergoes decomposition in the human intestines, breaking up into indol, skatol and phenol. The latter is carbolic acid. All these putrefactive acids from protein overconsumption irritate nerve endings and prolong pain. So I restricted our three middle-agers to no more than about two ounces of protein a day. Not only that, but because flesh proteins are often laden with toxic residue or chemical injectibles (stilbestrol, adrenalin, etc.) I confined these patients to pure, nontoxic protein in the form of wheat germ, soy beans, pecan nuts, and sunflower seeds.

In these cases the favorite among nuts is pecans. They are rich in pyridoxine, and this I have found stills pains in the body. Also, I urge the frequent use of brown rice because of its valuable content of pangamic acid, a useful ingredient in painful maladies.

Lastly, I had a special pain-reducing helper—garlic—for the three men, a great aid which all but the dentist adopted—the latter claiming he couldn't abide garlic because of working so closely with patients, a good enough reason. I refer to the technique of eating every night for two weeks an open-faced sandwich of peanut butter liberally sprinkled with a chopped-up clove or toe of garlic. The raw garlic thus is easily consumed, spread over the single slice of peanut-buttered bread. For reasons not clearly understood it takes some 14 days for this to show results; and it must be done at bedtime without interruption, for if a day is missed it appears that the entire program must be begun all over again.

PUTTING IT ALL TOGETHER

When treating people with painful arms or legs who engage in one-sided sports, I'd found that a real cure is virtually impossible unless they quit, or at least reverse, their one-sided activities.

In the aforementioned case of the dentist I had the greatest problem. Working sideways with his patients (and this applies to watchmakers and others with one-sided occupations), it was not enough merely to stop his tennis games. I had to X-ray his spine for the scoliotic curvature, something I dislike doing because of the carcinogenic (cancer-causing) propensities in the rays, and commence treatments to bring the vertebrae into alignment, thus removing the pressures on nerves that the X-rays revealed. If I had allowed tennis during the treatments, results would not be forthcoming or would be very slow in appearing; for instead of maintaining the benefits he obtained from treatments he would have lost the relief he'd gained every time he served a tennis ball with vigor over the net, forcing the poor painful leg into renewed strain through giant swings to one side.

When I put it all together I realize that it triggered a useful piece of research in that it told me that one-sided activities must be forbidden in cases of sciatica, sacroiliac, lumbosacral, lumbago and associated problems.

It may be all right for people in good health to participate in unilateral exercises such as bowling, golf, tennis, handball. I have reservations on this. But I am quite sure that people with ailments of *whatever* kind ought to confine themselves to bilateral sports and games.

I counsel people to exercise. Even cardiacs are given special exercises that I have devised for them. Everyone needs such activities if only to reoxygenate the body from time to time. But my preferences are for two-sided sports: rowing, bicycling or tricycling for elderly folk, volleyball games, vigorious walking strides, two-handed swimming strokes.

Inactivity *de*mineralizes human bones and makes fractures more easily possible. Activity *re*mineralizes bones. It is therefore not quite enough for oldsters merely to rock in their rocking chairs. Even for those with serious heart dysfunctions I've developed exercises that tend to build in some auxiliary tiny arteries that can feed the needed blood into the stricken heart area—these to be found in another section of this book.

In my own case, being an active lover of tennis, or squash, I play with two racquets. Yes, with two, actually. A newspaper in Mexico City ran a story of this once, accompanied with a photo of me playing with two racquets. The caption that accompanied this story and photo explained that I was "A doctor's doctor who taught that one side of the body should not be developed at the expense of the other, and therefore advised that all sports for humans should be two-sided or bilateral."

Chapter Fourteen

The Problem of the
After-Dinner Stroll

Are you concerned about a sallow complexion? Lifeless skin? Coated tongue?

Does everything you eat seem to turn to gas in your stomach? Is this one of your chief ailments? Do you suffer the embarrassment of manufacturing so much gas after you eat that friends chide you about being in competition with the gas company?

Associated with this are other conditions: belching, constipation, pimples and generally poor complexion.

Many who are beset by the above complaints are active, they exercise a great deal, they take *constitutional walks* after meals and do deep breathing while they walk.

But they need to get hold of one precious fact and observe it. The fact is that after eating a person ought to rest, take it easy, never become active.

Observe what the animals do. They play and romp *before* they eat. After their meal they curl up and nap.

It is bad for you to do otherwise. It may rob your digestive capacity of needed "blood-fuel" and bring on flatulence, bad breath, a coated tongue, a sallow complexion.

The reasons for this are made clear in the research story set forth in these next few pages.

***

A Research Appraisal of After-Dinner Strolls

The man told me a little conspiratorially that he must bring his wife into the office "because she needs a little lecture from you." In his opinion she was a "health nut" in the sense that she loved walking with vigorous strides even when he felt like slumping in his favorite easy chair. The way he told it, it appeared that he was right, that his wife did indeed need a bit of straightening out.

When I saw the lady I was surprised. Her legs were sturdy and her body seemed strong, but her complexion was sallow and sickish in appearance. The story was that her only complaint was "in the digestive department."

She was constipated. Everything she ate turned into gases, she said. It was embarrassing how often she couldn't help belching in public.

"How can this be, doctor?" she wanted to know. "I am active, not sedentary. Since my youth I've been athletic. I am a great walker. Even after every meal with my husband in the evening we take a long active walk."

That was it! She supplied the answer. It was an answer that triggered this particular adventure in research.

"You walk after your dinner—right after it?" I demanded. She nodded energetically, happy to answer in the affirmative. So she received the "little lecture" that her husband said she needed.

This was the story she got.

After one eats one should rest. It's a way of doing nothing *with intelligence.* Observe the animals. After they eat they curl up and nap.

Animals are not blessed with our pompous *scientificness.* They cannot analyze their affairs, so they listen to the wisdom of their bodies. After consuming a meal, the blood is needed in the organs of digestion. It's the fuel the digestive apparatus needs for "cooking down" the meal and reducing it to the normal end-products of digestion. When you walk after a meal you use the muscles of locomotion, and *they* also need blood for this. So what happens is that the muscles of *walking* pull some of the needed blood away from the *digesting* organs. The animals know this without being told. That's why they do not exercise after eating. But unlike animals, you do not *listen to the wisdom of your body!* So you do have to be told about it.

PUTTING IT ALL TOGETHER

It is not wise to listen to the advice of anyone to take an after-dinner stroll. My research has shown beyond any peradventure of doubt that activity following food-consumption makes for digestive problems. It is physiologically wrong. My advice is to allow the blood to be in the digestive organs after eating. There it is needed for thorough digestion of what you've consumed. If you walk too soon after a meal, the walking muscles will demand and get some of that blood for their own use. Do not divide your blood capacity that way. When I'd learned this bit of research wisdom and told it to patients, many achieved digestive health merely from stopping their after-dinner strolls because they were told that it's good "to walk the meal down." When walking, moreover, a casual stroll is nothing aside from getting some fresh air. When walking, I advise walking with vigor. Get the muscles to use a lot of blood when they work, not just a little.

Chapter Fifteen

A New Look at the Common Cold

I can declare without equivocation that a cure for the cold will never be found. The doctors are barking up the wrong tree.

Why? How do I know?

Here's why and how. The reason why a cure for the common cold will never be found is that the cold itself *is* the cure.

Think about it a minute yourself to sort out the facts and logic of this. Try to understand what there is about the common cold that makes it a cure rather than a sickness.

Then keep reading.

***

The Common Cold: Why a Cure Is Impossible

The little blonde doll of a girl sat in my office sniffling and dabbing her tearing eyes with paper towels. Her distressed mother told me of her tendency toward colds. She was never without a cold it seemed. It was a cross the child had to bear. "Last summer," the mother said, "we even gave her shots all those months to prevent these attacks—and now look at her."

This was the kind of recitation that made me bristle. My own former researches had told me that there is *no* cure for the common cold because *the cold itself IS the cure!*

The cold is the organism's way of opening the safety valves to save itself from an overload of accumulated poisons. It is the expression of the body's built-in safeguards against an inimical environment.

You Sneeze Your Cold Away

The system is overstuffed or poisoned, it is full of accumulated wastes that make function difficult. So the *common cold* is nature's *common way* of relieving itself and saving itself. A final straw such as foul air or a cold wind tips the scales and the safety mechanism, which is the cold, gets to work. The victim sneezes out the debris. The clogged nose empties the body of excess mucus. A fever burns up (oxidizes) the toxic pile-up. A sweating period opens a million pores and excretes the harmful accumulations by that route.

Any medicine for a cold is a suppressive agent. The cold itself is the cure—curing the body, cleansing it, preparing it for a healthy thereafter. It is unbelievable nonsense—which means *no* sense—and incredibly unscientific to pollute a human bloodstream with shots, as was done in the innocent child before me. The body subject to colds already has enough burdens to deal with; now the medical "scientists" load the blood with more pollutants that the blood will need to labor to filter out.

PUTTING IT ALL TOGETHER

If you have a cold, *do nothing intelligently.* Listen to the wisdom of the body. With a cold the appetite wanes. Don't eat. When an animal is sick it curls up and rests, doing nothing. You do the same.

Do nothing at all until the body has *cured itself.* All the aid you can offer intelligently is to free the nerve lines of pressures if any exist. Get on your hands and knees and sway down as far as possible, then arch up as far as possible. Walk on all fours. Rest in the counter-gravity, knee-chest position. If you need activity, run a race with yourself or someone else on your hands and knees. This tends to align the spine and eliminate vertebral misalignments.

Chapter Sixteen

Exploring the Sunbath
—and Your Shadow

How would you like to take all the sunbaths you want and never suffer a bit of harm or after-pain?

It can be done—easily.

If sunshine is your nemesis, but you at the same time like the looks of a suntan on your skin, you can heave a sigh of relief. Now it is possible to shake off the old enemy of sunburn and still achieve your heart's desire.

It all hinges on a simple thing: Just measure the length of your shadow.

Yes, your shadow. Stand on the beach or in the middle of a yard where nothing will interfere with your ability to see your shadow. Now compare your own height with the length of the shadow cast by your body. If the shadow that you cast is longer than you are tall, that's a safe time to be out in the sun. Usually you will find the shadow like this before ten in the morning and after four in the afternoon.

But if the shadow of your body is *shorter* than you are tall, it means that the rays are coming down dangerously straight and sharp, not on a slanted plane as they are in early morning and late afternoon, and in straight downward sharpness the rays may give you dangerous serum poisoning and even worse.

The whole story is within the little project described in the next few pages.

***

The Sun and Your Shadow

The young, blond Adonis was a foolish sun-worshiper. He hadn't the protective integument in his skin for that. But he loved darkening his skin with the sun's rays, even darkening the natural cornsilk color of his hair to a muddy brown.

At first his nose merely peeled. Then he blistered. At last he was self-dosed with ultra-violet poisoning. This was caught in time. I have seen it so severe as to be fatal.

At the time I had a habit of inviting clinic patients once a month to an evening lecture. The idea was to give them a chance to ask hanging questions that I may have been too rushed to answer during the busy daytime schedule. After this harrowing sunburn case with the blond sun idolizer I asked the assembled patients about their sunbathing habits.

Not a single person in the room knew how to deal with the sun. They had no idea about the how or when of correct, beneficial sunbathing. It started up a little research project in my office, and thereafter I kept tabs on how people used—and abused—the sun.

The net results, and my instructions to patients, were as follows.

Sunshine is good and useful. It gives you a free meal of vitamin D. It is good for the bones, protects against colds, benefits the metabolic processes, enhances healing mechanisms in the body, and promotes good sleep. But all this is true only when the sunshine is absorbed between the hours of, say, 8 to 10 in the morning and after 4 in the afternoon. Why so? Here's why.

After 10:00 a.m. the sun is high overhead, its rays slant straight down and are wickedly intense. They burn, blister, give you an overdose of ultra-violet rays—more than the body can absorb or utilize. This is toxic for the organism; it can be a deadly poison. This condition lasts until about 4:00 in the afternoon. Before 10:00 in the morning and after 4:00 in the afternoon, however, the sun is either rising or waning. Its rays are slanted obliquely rather than straight down, thus less powerful and less inclined to burn the tissues. The natural oils of the skin will promote photosynthesis and the beneficial rays will convert into good vitamin D. For this reason one should not wash or shower just before sunbathing, thus washing off the body oils, and not shower right after a sunbath and thus wash away the oils while conversion to vitamin D is still going on.

PUTTING IT ALL TOGETHER

Your body casts a shadow in the sunshine. The best test for sunbathing safety is in the length of your shadow. In the early morning and late afternoon the oblique rays will make the shadow longer than you are tall. That's the safe period for taking your sunbath.

Between ten and four the sun's rays are too straight for your good and the shadow cast by the sun will be shorter than you are tall. Stand in the middle of your sunbathing area, in your back yard or beach area where nothing obstructs the rays, and note the shadow. If it is taller than your height, okay. If it's shorter than your height, keep away. Even when walking in the sun during such hours, wear a head covering. The men in the tropics aren't altogether stupid with their protective, wide-brimmed sombreros, you know.

Chapter Seventeen

The Question of High Protein Diets

Do you suspect that you are toxic?

Do you have the feeling that your inner plumbing is not as clean and functional as it ought to be?

Or have you gone headlong and enthusiastically into the widely recommended high protein diet? And has anything happened to cause you to suspect that it is making you ill rather than well?

It may be that on a *low* protein diet you can more surely and safely lose all that toxicity, and that bothersome flatulence, and those skin rashes attributable to poor elimination.

You must forgive this seeming indelicacy, but one dependable test of a protein diet is the odor of your stools. Yes, that's the way to determine all by yourself whether you are consuming an "overdose" of proteins daily. If the odor that lingers in the bathroom after a BM is strong and foul, that's the measuring stick. It means that you have fed yourself more proteins than the body can handle.

The evidence is that the surplus protein which the organism is unable to reduce down to the normal end-products of digestion has decomposed into acids. They are smelly acids called indol, skatol, and phenol (carbolic) acid.

Very indelicate, I agree. But I mean this to be an informative and beneficial book rather than a social club, and these things are altogether true and important to know.

If you agree, then more of it is explained in the following pages and I urge you to read on.

***

Arresting Research with High Protein Diets

Long ago, way back in the beginning of my doctoring career, I suspected that people were consuming too much protein. I was suspicious of the "official handouts," fearing they were influenced by the dairy industry and/or powerful meat associations.

What caused me to doubt the value of a high protein intake was originally a good bit of reading on the subject, then a spate of original research control tests.

Sherman of Columbia, who'd written the definitive work on diet used by just about every student nurse in a nursing school, said that no human could utilize more than *70 grams* of protein. Chittendon of Yale, another giant in research, found in his many researching years that even Olympic athletes, with their great bursts of energy, could not fully utilize as little as *50 grams* of protein—which means that some of those 50 grams they consumed were excreted, unutilized, through bowels and kidneys. McCollum of Johns Hopkins discovered that he could induce cancer and nephritis (Bright's disease) in rats only on a high protein diet, never on a low one.

Seventy grams, fifty grams—how much is that? Roughly counting 29 grams to the ounce, it means that humans cannot use much more that two ounces of protein in one day. That's pure protein. Your 8-ounce steak of lean beef contains just about that much. But in my research I found that patients were consuming that much and more just for lunch. Besides, they had bacon or ham for breakfast. Eggs in addition, making more of a protein intake. Then came the evening meal with a really whopping helping of meat or cheese or milk or fish or nuts. Beans and other protein vegetables on top of that. And since all foods, almost without exception, contain *some* content of protein, they were ingesting enough of the stuff for a quartet of men.

"But I need protein for my strength," they said. "Doc says to eat lots and lots of protein—it protects me."

"Oh?" I often *oh'd* back at them, raising an eyebrow. "Where do you think the strong-as-a-horse *horse* gets its strength on that puny low protein diet it consumes? And the ox? Wouldn't you like to be strong as an ox? And the elephant— also on a very low protein intake!"

The Body Cannot Metabolize High Protein Diets

No wonder these people were sick. Flatulent. Toxic to a high degree. Constipated. Suffering skin rashes and other signs of insufficient elimination, such as foul breath. All excess intake of protein had to turn into toxic debris. Not just *could* putrefy— but *had* to. The body is able to store an excess of fatty foods or starches or sugars; people who overeat on them just get stout. But the body has no capability at all to store protein beyond its daily needs. What isn't utilized in daily cell-rebuilding and the like must—not just may but *must*—decompose in the human intestines into three stinky, toxic acids: indol, skatol and phenol (which is carbolic acid). That's why human stool matter smells foul—whereas the manure or excretions of low-protein-consuming animals isn't stinky in the same way at all!

What They Say is True But Not the Whole Truth Do They Say

The warning is that we cannot live without protein. This is correct. Without a daily ration of protein foodstuffs to repair the bodily damages sustained by normal metabolic processes, the body will deteriorate and sicken. The starches and fats and other food items cannot do the job of proteins. Only proteins can rebuild the torn-down and worn-out tissue cells.

But to say you can't live without proteins is not the same as saying that you must have a high protein intake to live and be well and strong.

In a way—big surprise—the opposite is true! To put the matter epigrammatically, what they say is true but not the whole truth do they say. One sure way to get sick seems to be to eat an overload of protein.

There has been evidence, observed and compiled in Russia, that while an excess of protein often gives the illusion of *feeling better*, it is because the protein overload forces the bodily machinery to work harder and faster. It appears that the speed with which the organism utilizes and excretes its substances in protein metabolism is *the speed at which the body grows older.*

If you consume a high protein load of foodstuffs you may be unwittingly "using yourself up" more rapidly. I intend to keep a sharp eye out for further reports from the Russian Traumatology Institute.

PUTTING IT ALL TOGETHER

Cut down your daily intake of protein. My experience with geriatric cases especially makes this advice valid. When I advised older patients to restrict their intake of meat, fish, nuts, eggs and other proteins to something like two ounces a day they seemed to improve in health, almost without regard to what their problem was. Among the favored proteins are wheat germ (if not rancid), sunflower seeds or walnuts, avocado, coconut, on occasion a small helping of cottage cheese, and an egg on lesser occasions.

Chapter Eighteen

Studying the Skins
of Fruits and Vegetables

Have you ever been worried about "inside" trouble because you spotted undigested tomato skins in your stool matter?

And are you one of the many who don't like apple skin and potato peelings and the like, but eat the things religiously anyway as a duty to health because "they say" that that's the healthiest part of the food?

If you dislike skins, skip them. You may just be doing yourself a favor at the same time.

In support of this position, take a look at the research project hereinafter described.

***

An Adventure with Fruit Skins: To Eat or Not to Eat

A patient asked a simple question. "Why do I always find undigested tomato skins in the stools?"

I remembered that I had seen the same thing myself. Also, I recalled the skins of corn niblets failed to undergo complete digestion and escaped from the bowel whole.

The researcher in my make-up was aroused. Was it possible that the human body did not manufacture enzymes strong enough to break down fruit skins?

Weren't they meant to be eaten?

Simply because we'd always been told that *the best part was in the skin,* did that absolutely make it so?

The investigation began. The research was conducted on a broad scale. Here are my findings.

Tracing back, it must have been the illustrious McCollum of Johns Hopkins who started it with his potato peelings for sailors severely ill because they had been on shipboard for months without fresh vegetables or fruits.

Since then, doctors have said that the best part of any fruit's or vegetable's nutritional value is in the skin. Especially was this so, they declared, when it related to vitamin and mineral content.

Their mistake was that they *imagined* the sailors were fed *only* potato skins whereas they were given thick cuttings of potato slices near the skin, and including the skin. Furthermore, the skin of the potato is not as impermeable as the skin of the apple, tomato, etc.

Skins are air-tight and water-tight. They are impermeable envelopes containing the inner nutritional goodies.

They were not meant to be consumed!

We do not have the enzymes in the body to digest apple skins or tomato skins, for example, clear down to their normal end-products of digestion. This is why one notices whole, undigested tomato skins in the stools. A better scientific case can be made for the middle of the fruit to be the best part. It is in the middle where the seeds are. Those seeds in the center of fruits are the life factors of the fruits. The life and goodness of each fruit originally came from the seeds in each fruit.

The life is in the seeds. The seeds are in the center of the fruit. Ergo: the best parts of fruits are the centers of fruits.

PUTTING IT ALL TOGETHER

I advise people to peel apples, tomatoes, other fruits and all "peelable" vegetables just as they do oranges and bananas. It is unwise, of course, to peel deeply into the fruit or vegetable, for the part removed should be as thin as possible. If tomatoes are first thrust into very hot water, which expands them, and then dipped quickly into cold water to shrink the skin, peeling becomes an easy matter. Except for seedless grapes, I advise that grape skins should not be consumed. They contain purple compounds of tannin, a constipating element. Also corn and beans should be soaked until the outer impermeable skin-envelopes come away.

Chapter Nineteen

The Best Time for Exercise

If you are a poor sleeper you will want to know what is written here.

If you are an older person with an ever-present fear of fracturing your bones, or if you are a shallow breather who feels that there is never quite enough oxygen in his lungs, then the little experiment recounted next may have special meaning for you.

Most doctors who are worth their salt tell us to do *some* exercise. But how many have ever told us *when* it's best to exercise? This is a matter they appear not to have researched at all.

But now it can be told. You can hug the truth to your breast and inscribe it ineradicably in the memory by way of a little rhyming sentence.

"What you gain at bedtime you retain during bedtime."

When do you suppose that body of yours gets a chance to heal and repair its damaged parts? It isn't when you are working and straining, but when you are quiescent and at restful ease. Thus the benefits of exercising just before you retire are there to benefit your body all through the hours in bed when you aren't prancing around. During sleep the respirations slow down, metabolic processes take over in a serious uninterrupted way, and the healing mechanisms of the organism proceed apace.

I recommend that you carefully read the following research item. Once read, its benefits will serve you throughout your life—and you will yearn to share them with others.

***

A Researcher Finds the Best Time to Exercise

Many patients who like to exercise say they are too lazy or sleepy to do any exercising at bedtime.

This is understandable. Yet it falls on me to consider the physiological and neurological sides of the question. It may be a bit awkward to do some improvement drills before going to sleep, but when is exercise *most useful* for the organism?

When we look at it that way, the very best time to give the body a special workout is at bedtime. Just as some acts on TV believe in audience-participation, I believe in patient-participation. When my patient understands fully *why* he is instructed to do anything, he participates with me in the project, usually with enthusiasm as well as understanding.

I tried it out as a little research program, advising the office patients to exercise at different times of the day. Now I believe in exercise—moderate and regular exercise—even for the very elderly. My researches showed that exercising oldsters hardly ever fractured their bones when they fell, for the exercise programs nourished their bones with minerals and gave them both hardness and suppleness or resiliency. But since many old persons are poor sleepers, the researches showed that those with insomnia also slept better when they exercised at bedtime.

I obtained the same finding for younger people. In running it down, the reasons came to hand. It was incredible that the matter had not been researched before—the reasons were so sensible and right.

Exercise is most beneficial just before retiring because of this: *What you gain at bedtime you maintain during bedtime.* This applies especially to breathing exercises such as the diaphragm drill and the rib-widening effort, for they oxygenate the entire system. With better oxygenation one not only sleeps better but his system repairs the damages of the day more efficiently. Breath, not bread, is the staff of life.

Although exercise can be profitable at all times of the day, and I advise it for mornings and afternoons also in most cases, the study I conducted showed conclusively that it was best at the retiring hour. It does not apply, however, to wildly energetic exercises that can stimulate one into wakefulness.

Healing and bodily repairs go on while you are lying recumbent, not while upright and active. Daytimes you heave and strain, and twist and turn, and sustain stresses and bodily impacts. It is when these strains on the organsim are absent, while lying quietly in bed, that the metabolic processes slow down, respirations become deeper and less rapid and the body rejuvenates itself for the next day. The damages of the workaday world cannot be repaired by the body's self-healing forces during your active hours. Therefore exercise is most beneficial at bedtime because its benefits last during the hours when your weight is off your feet and the body is healing itself.

PUTTING IT ALL TOGETHER

Do not forego exercising mornings and at all other times when you like to exercise. But do not forget to do *some* exercises at bedtime. Stand in front of an open window, raise your arms and part your lips, then pant like a dog pants. This moves and exercises the diaphragm. Get on your hands and knees and sway your backbone into a deep hollow, then arch upward to the greatest height possible, repeating several times. Stand and think of your lower ribs and consciously separate them, widen them. This is your best exercise at the best time.

Chapter Twenty

Advice for a Food Worrier

If you are a food worrier, this is for you.

If, moreover, you frequent the health food stores and pay far more for your foods than you would at regular markets *but are still sickish*—and you never seem to improve in any solid way despite your attention to "the best foods," then you ought to fairly vibrate to this particular research story.

Why do you not almost immediately improve and get well when you buy and consume foods that are known to be potentially health-building?

Ah, there's a real, deep-down explanation there.

"The potential value of any food is not its actual value."

Would you believe it? I ask you to re-read what is written above in quotation marks.

If you are skinny and cannot gain weight; if you are stout and cannot lose weight even though you consistently undereat; if you are constipated, or lack in energy, then you need to know that your organism is probably not able to *convert* properly what you eat. It cannot convert the *potential* value of what you eat into *actual* value.

And now, in the pages ahead, you will learn why—and what to do about it.

***

Why Good Food Doesn't Always Mean Good Health

The young lady was very well read and also very athletic. She walked with a rapid stride, was always buoyant and happy, her ice-blue eyes full of twinkles. And she said without apology that she was "a health nut."

When I complimented her on being "full of life" she said that she was also "full of bones"—far too bony for her happiness. And she was right. Her face had a peaches-and-cream complexion, her hair was a beautiful straw yellow which went well with those sharp blue eyes, but she was skinny as a beanpole with her collarbones and ribs sticking out to be counted.

"That's why I'm here," she complained. "I've got to put a little more flesh onto this skeleton of mine. Why can't I?"

It developed that because she was a self-acclaimed "health nut," she bought most of her foods in the health food stores. Only the best for her. No artificial colorings or flavorings. No carcinogens in any food item. Organically grown vegetables.

"I read the labels on packages and cans," she insisted. "I pay twice for a lot of foods that are cheaper in supermarkets. My energy is fine and I feel reasonably good. But there are two things, Doctor Morrison. Even though I'm careful to buy and eat only the best foods, I'm forever constipated. And even though I never allow poorly combined foods to enter my mouth, I can't gain an ounce."

Why Food Worriers Stay Sick

She was making an all-too-common error of health enthusiasts. I recall that her comments started up a research project that confirmed what I am now about to say. The great truth is this: *The potential value of any food is not its actual value.*

Please read that last sentence again. Read it many times and memorize it. Just because a certain food is potentially valuable for the human system, it is not of actual value until it is absorbed. Absorbed and converted. Converted and utilized. Utilized and appropriated. Appropriated by the system as good cells and tissues: good bone cells, muscle cells, gland cells, etc.

Our blonde, springy, alert "health nut" was not alert to the fact that she had a large number of nerve pressures in her spine. She was not alert to the fact that these pressures interfered with the free flow of digestive energy in the form of nerve impulses to the digestive organs. Without the energizing and function-directing impulses, the organs could not possibly perform the digesting job they were intended to perform—any more than a motor could work properly if not plugged into its source of energy.

What needed to be done was a simple thing to do by anyone trained as I was trained. I removed the pressure interference on the nerve pathways as they emanated from the spine. With the offending vertebrae again in correct alignment, the nerve impulses again could flow through to the digestive organs without being pinched off or interfered with. When once the digestive *power was turned on*, our pretty lady had the digestive capacity to reduce down her food intake to their normal end-products. The system then used the food properly and completely. The potential in her good food items was there. Now, with a full and free flow of energy and directional signals to her organs of digestion, the system *converted potential food value into actual value.*

No drugs or shots or surgery could have taken those offending nerve pressures away. Mere *good foods* were not good enough to ensure good appropriation of the values inherent in those foods.

The potential value of any food is not its actual value.

To be changed from potential to actual value the food item—even the very best food item—must be first absorbed, converted, utilized, appropriated by the system.

Researching this matter I discovered that all patients with digestive problems had pressures on nerves that served their digestive organs. There were no exceptions. All the strains and stresses of a physical nature in their lifetime forced or jolted spinal vertebrae out of position, and these pinched the nerves, preventing the flow of digestive power to the organs served by such nerves.

This was why skinny people who "ate only the best foods" couldn't improve and couldn't gain an ounce. It was also why the chronically constipated or dyspeptic cases who similarly "bought only the best foods and carefully avoided incompatible food combinations" remained ill and complaining. They had spinal nerve pressures, I found, and until the pathways to their digestive organs were cleared of pressures they hadn't the digestive power to convert even good foods into good health.

PUTTING IT ALL TOGETHER

No matter how potentially good a food you consume is, if your system lacks the capacity or nerve power to appropriate it, it is as though you hadn't eaten it. To make potentially valuable foods actually valuable to your organism, see that the nerves to your digestive organs are not blocked, pinched, interfering with the conductivity of digestive power to the stomach, pancreas, liver. At bedtime each day you should perform the *nerve-unpinching exercises and drills* given in Chapter Thirty-One. If very badly constipated or lacking in digestive capacity, do the drills several times a day. If necessary, get a chiropractic doctor to start the spine alignment process for you, then take it up *and keep it up* on your own.

If very stout and you cannot lose weight even though you do not overeat, it may be that the nerves to the endocrines are blocked, in which case the nerve-unpinching drills will *turn on the power* to the ductless glands. If you eat fresh fruits and green and good proteins such as wheat germ and sunflower seeds and still ail, then it may easily be that your system is not converting potential values into actual food values. See to opening the pinched nerve lines, then see the vast health difference it makes.

Chapter Twenty-One

A Secret About Exercise

Is your memory faulty?

Are you a cardiac victim, or a cardiac cripple, or have you been told that you're on the way to having a heart attack if you don't change your ways?

And now—a big question. Have you ever thought that all the advice you've heard about exercise may be wrong? Wrong— that is—if it advised you to stand or sit up and do the various exercising routines.

Why so? Because of the soundest reasons, reasons you immediately will recognize as correct even if you are not a doctor.

The main reason is that when you stand or sit during exercise you accelerate the heart action to pump blood *uphill*. The key there is uphill. To be good to your heart and blood vessels you have to send blood circulating to the oxygen-starved cells throughout the body *on the level*, not upstairs to the neck and head against gravity.

This is not difficult to understand. Yet it has not been grappled with properly in all these years by the healing or doctoring professions.

For you to understand it more fully—and become greatly benefited thereby—please read and heed the words that follow.

***

Researching the Relative Value of Upright and Horizontal Exercise

I have had many experiences with elderly male patients who enjoyed doing daily excercises. Some did the exercises for sheer pleasure, others because they wanted physical fitness. Relatively few women were as dedicated to daily exercise programs as their male counterparts.

To indulge the elderly patients, I would let them tell me in detail about their prowess on the exercise field or carpet at home. They did so many push-ups, this many knee bends, that many elephant swings. But often they would stop mid-way in the recitations, forgetting what they wanted to say. They had memory lapses. Signs of hardening of the arteries were evident.

One day a thought came to me out of the seeming nowhere. Why so much arteriosclerosis in those who exercised? Why the forgetfulness they evidenced, those embarrassing lapses in memory? Wasn't the brain getting enough blood to oxygenate the peripheral tissues?

I was off on one of my "smallish" adventures in research.

To the man who had hardening of the arteries the loss of memory was not a *smallish* matter; it was one of great and grave concern. Just the same, to me it was small in the sense that it was easy to run down to sensible, physiologically documentable conclusions. His memory often failed because the littlest vessels in the brain were not sufficiently large to transport the blood needed to nourish the brain with oxygen. They weren't large enough because not enough of the blood which carried the oxygen could get through to those brain vessels, notably what we label the circle of Willis. His assiduous exercise program, in fact, might be hurting rather than helping the condition.

Don't Exercise Against Gravity

This was because he did his exercises standing or sitting. *They were done against gravity.* The blood had to push its load of vital oxygen straight uphill to those already small-and-hardened arteries.

But what if he did his exercising in the horizontal position!

What if he occasionally exercised with his head lower than his body? Suppose I instructed him to do *all* his drills and movements lying on his back, or on his abdomen, or in the knee-chest position, or crosswise on a bed with his head hanging down a bit? Then the blood would flow to those oxygen-impoverished arterioles with ease. The flow would be downhill. It would be following gravity, not fighting it. The heart would not be laboring to force those big gobs of blood straight uphill some 72 times every minute. Then the undernourished brain vessels would get nourished, thinking would become clearer, and memory lapses would tend to slow down or disappear.

PUTTING IT ALL TOGETHER

The heart is unstrained when it works on a level plane. Do all exercises in a horizontal position. Lie on your chest and make believe you are doing the breast stroke of swimmers. Lie on your back and spin your legs around in one direction and in reverse, as though riding a bicycle upside down forward and backward. Get on your knees and chest and in that position, head slightly down, open the lips and pant like a dog, thus exercising the diaphragm for improved oxygenation. Lie crosswise on a bed, head hanging over the edge a bit, and bring the knees vigorously to the chest, thus spreading apart the lower spinal vertebrae and helping to position the pelvis properly. Devise other exercises to your taste in the straight-across (horizontal) rather than the upside-uphill (vertical) position.

If you are a cardiac victim or suffer from hardening of the arteries, this is especially important. Vigorous exercises in the standing up-and-down position force the heart to pump upward. The heart thus may dilate unduly, causing it damage. The vessels also are forced to expand, not made to expand naturally as when gravity favors you. This risks a possible aneurism—a possible blow-out. Try a mere week of doing all your exercising only in the horizontal position. Just see if that one week of physiologically logical and correct positioning doesn't make you want to exclaim, "Now why didn't somebody tell me this before!"

Chapter Twenty-Two

A Restudy of Milk

It is probably true that the last advertisement about milk to cross your path said, "No one ever outgrows the need for milk."

If you felt inclined to believe this, I ask you to consider the following points.

1. Milk is mainly a protein food.
2. The human body is constructed in such a way that proteins are absolutely necessary to the maintenance of health.
3. But protein food must be chewed. The body has no capacity to handle proteins unchewed.
4. Depending on milk as so many do, one would think that there's an insufficiency of proteins around—what with nuts, cheese, wheat germ, many grains, beans, fish, eggs, meat and many protein-rich vegetables.
5. There is no known way to chew milk in the way that proteins must be chewed. As a liquid, milk is of course swallowed in gulps. The calf takes the same kind of milk that you drink from its Mama Cow drop by drop, not in gulps. The human baby at the mother's breast suckles milk also drop by drop.
6. Any wonder that half the complaints that pediatricians attend to flow from infant illnesses, changing formulas and watering down milk with nonmilk products to eliminate baby ailments?

Interesting?
What follows is even more so.

***

A Reassessment of Milk: Proteins Must Always Be Chewed

It is well known that advertising copy often assures us most soothingly that what is actually harmful for us is truly great and healthful.

The advertising connected with milk almost falls in this class. "You can never outgrow your need for milk," go some of the ads. This kind of ad wants you to think that milk is always and forever good for you. Well, it isn't. There are plenty of valid, sound, really scientific arguments against milk. So we must warily approach the beautiful advertising that assures us of the mis-fact that "Milk is nature's most perfect food."

Rubbish!

Perfect for whom? Cow's milk may be perfect for the calf. When the human being has developed teeth with which to chew more substantial fare, it is nature's signal that he must go to solid foods. Milk also lacks iodine and iron—thus, it is not anything like perfect. If the mother who unwittingly feeds her baby on cow's milk thinking it is just great and perfect, as the ads say, didn't supplement the bovine milk with orange juice and something like cod liver oil she'd have a sicker baby on her hands than she now usually has.

I mean to spell out a number of objections to milk in this section of the book. I must warn unknowing persons about the real, unmentioned effects of pasteurization. About the mucus-forming effects of milk which endanger those with emphysema, asthma and lung or bronchial problems or tendencies. About *overproteinizing* the body as a distinct possibility when milk is used. About the harmfulness of crossing the species; for what the human being should use is human milk, what the calf needs is the mother-cow's milk, not milk from goats or human females. But most of all I wish to stress the following danger of milk.

Protein should be chewed. It should be taken in solid form. The human body has no proper provision for handling protein that is thrown down the gullet like water thrown down the radiator of one's car. The enzyme in the stomach that is there to begin digesting protein food items just cannot COPE with a gusher of fluid protein that hits it all at once like a torrent. It can cope well only with protein that comes down the esophagus little by little, drop by drop—protein, that is, which is chewed, macerated and masticated in the mouth, properly prepared for it before it is sent down to the stomach.

How do I know that this is true? That all this exact and specific information is scientific and physiologically sound? Because it has proved to be true in tests among milk-drinking patients. It went through all the pragmatic hurdles and passed all pragmatic tests. When I instructed those with digestive and patently overproteinized symptoms (gas, foul stools, bad breath, etc.), who mistakenly consumed quantities of milk daily, to change completely to chewable protein items such as nuts or even grains, they all improved to some extent. If they held the chewable protein intake down to reasonable proportions—say no more than two ounces a day—they improved even more; certainly more than those who believed the medical misinformation that everyone needs a high protein diet.

Louis Pasteur didn't even think of milk when he devised the partial heating method that is now called pasteurization. It was his technique for keeping wine from going sour. It works that way because when a fluid is heated for half an hour at 62 degrees Centigrade (143° F.) the organic life in the fluid is stabilized. It's preserved. It no longer has the living vitality of an unheated article of food. Just as the heat kills the pathogenic bacteria in milk—most bacteria but by no means all, let it be known—it kills the living vitality of the food also. Therefore the calcium content of milk, for which milk is drunk *specifically* by many persons, becomes in a way inappropriable calcium. It cannot be properly and fully and beneficially utilized by the system. Its relation to the magnesium factor is altered, rendered unbalanced, made unutilizable.

I do not fully agree with natural living enthusiasts that cooked food is dead food. In many cases this is true; but it is overblown and not true in some cases. In the case of milk, however, I must agree that heated milk becomes in a metabolic sense dead, or almost dead, food.

Everyone Outgrows His Need for Milk

The milk people advertise with pride that their product has a such-and-such *high* cream content. The higher the content of cream in the milk, the greater their pride and the better the milk, *they say*. But it is just this cream factor that is most harmful in milk. It is mucus forming in the human system. Persons, and especially children, with tendencies toward cold, bronchial coughs, nasal and throat phlegm formations, heavy mucus-laden chests, nearly all do better when milk is abandoned altogether. If milk is to be employed at all, I would certainly change to skimmed milk, particularly that with all of the cream removed.

Milk does not contain any appreciable amount of vitamin C, perfect though it is advertised to be. Pasteurization does a complete job of killing all of its vitamin D, which is why dairies advertise that their milk product is "fortified" with vitamin D. First their heating process cooks the vitamin out, then the natural stuff is supplanted with their own synthetic "fortified" variety.

Do you want a list of milk-related ailments in the human species? Well, the specific maladies directly traceable to milk consumption are, first of all, *allergies,* which alone should tell us that the system does not want this food. Heart diseases and attacks have also been traced to the use of milk. Also diarrhea, bodily weaknesses due to iron deficiency, chronic and systemic cramps, stomach irritations due to the fact that the protein in cow's milk differs from the protein in human milk. Many cases of milk-related skin rashes (eczema) and bloated stomachs, and arthritic joint pains, and asthma, nasal congestion, ear infections and even persistent vomiting, have been recorded. All this applies to some extent also to milk-derived products such as butter and cheese.

Besides the aforementioned faults of milk, it must be borne in mind that what one drinks from the milk bottle or carton is not from the same cow. It is from a large variety of cows, most likely, all collected in enormously vast receptacles and well mixed in the process. I submit that even if milk were acceptable it would have to be from the same animal, not a collection from a whole herd of beasts.

PUTTING IT ALL TOGETHER

To be well, you must chew all your protein-bearing foods. Milk cannot be chewed, thus it cannot make for good health. Also, the tendency is to overuse milk; that is, one tends to consume an oversupply of protein by drinking milk. As indicated elsewhere in this book (Chapter Twenty), anything more than two ounces of pure protein taken daily must undergo decomposition in the intestines and form harmful acids. It is advised that you should *never* use milk as a thirst quencher—in this area it is the worst of possible choices. Those with tendencies to colds and coughs should especially avoid the use of milk.

Chapter Twenty-Three

Examining the Primate Diet

Sometimes, when you have gone to doctor after doctor and nothing seems to help, don't you feel lost and baffled and kind of drifting on a vast sea without a thing to anchor to?

I ask you to believe a rare and beautiful truth. When all the doctors are baffled, your body isn't. It isn't baffled. It knows what to do. It knows how to heal that wound of yours, mend that gouged area, repair those scraped knees.

When you place tomato or corn seeds into the ground they always cone up tomatoes or corn, never raspberries or pumpkins. That's because the ground—or nature—is never baffled. It knows how to sort things out and knows what to do.

When you've cut your hand the body repairs the cut with skin cells, not bone cells. If your arm is broken the long brachium or ulna is cemented and bridged with bone cells, never liver or kidney cells.

In the body, when you are sick and don't seem to improve, hold on. The saying is that when you have come to the end of your rope tie a knot in it and hang on. I have found one sensible and exact way to let the body sort out the problems, get un-baffled, and do the right thing.

That one best way is the Primate Diet. It is the best and safest and most dependable way I have ever discovered.

Better find out about this Primate Diet. Here it is all set forth: both the research project behind it and the diet itself.
***

Researching a Perfectly Safe Health Haven—The Primate Diet

The body knows what is the matter even when the doctor is baffled and doesn't know. This is a tricky item to understand. It's so simple that it's a difficulty for educated minds to grasp. You have a cough or a skin eruption. Does the healing wait until the doctor has called the cough bronchitis or the eruption eczema? Or does the ailment begin at once to mend itself? The body, you see, knows what's the matter. And the body knows what to do for what's the matter. All the body asks is that you remove the obstructions to self-healing.

In my researches I have discovered three principal obstructive bulls-on-the-track. Here they are, all obstructing the body's ability to heal itself.

Three Major Causes of Illness

Number one is nerve pressure. Everyone twists and turns and falls and strains. Everyone accumulates pressures on various nerve lines. Then the organs served by such nerve lines are deprived of two items: functional power and healing power. So nerve pressures must be corrected, removed, unblocked. The drills in Chapter Thirty-One will show you how to do this. In dire cases, ask a chiropractic doctor to get the process started, then carry on alone from there. Nerve pressures constitute the chief killer of man. I do not believe that coronary occlusion is the nation's number one killer. Number one is pressure on nerves to the heart that make coronary occlusions possible.

Number two is drugs. All of them assault the organism and whip the already sick body into greater sickness. It's like whipping a tired horse. Of course the weary horse will make a last valiant effort under the lash of the whip. But at what cost to his energy reserves? Being thus whipped into unnatural bursts of energy, in the way that drugs stimulate unnatural functional efforts, the horse can drop dead without warning. The tragedy is that drugs *seem* to do something. And they really do. They swap symptoms, as Alexis Carrel noted. They divert what was visible into something else. Meanwhile the stomach cramps or the cough (or whatever) subside, and who knows or cares what is happening to start up a severe kidney disease!

Number three is one's food intake. Too much food and bad combinations of food obstruct the body's ability to mend its own damages. So what is one to do? Is there anything to do? I repeat what was written at the outset of this little adventure in research. Yes, there is a wonderfully effective and wholly safe thing to do, a program that will not obstruct healing.

Go on fruits for a week. Easy enough? Does it sound too simplistic? Well, eat only fruits for just one week and see for yourself.

Man is a *primate*. (See Thomas Henry Huxley's "Man's Place in Nature.") What does a primate eat? With the rarest of exceptions, only fruits. It is fruit that is the *natural* food for mankind, for all primates. Long before man wandered from his tropical beginnings and had to adapt to vegetarianism, he was a *fruitarian*. I need not trace the evolutionary steps that all educated persons know: First the primate ate only fruits; then when fruits were not abundant in colder climates he adapted to vegetables; finally in very cold northerly wanderings where all vegetation was sparse but hunting and fishing was at hand he adapted to flesh foods.

So, back to our main theme. If sick and baffled by your sickness, send away the doctor and take charge of yourself. Go back to primal beginnings, and that will give the entire organism a chance to mend itself. Go back to fruits exclusively. Doing this, you'll be going back to source. You will be giving your body a chance to right itself.

PUTTING IT ALL TOGETHER

When no one else knows what is the matter with your ailing body, the body knows. Doctors and you may be perplexed, but the body knows what the ailment is and knows how to repair it. Try eating fruits alone for one test week. You cannot do damage in just one week of testing this way. See what miracles can happen. For your own safety remember that the body makes all its own necessary drugs. All the hormones you need and can use. All your needed insulin, adrenalin, pepsin, hydrochloric acid, cortisone, enzymes, the lot. The body does this if you do not obstruct it in its functions or if, being obstructed, you remove the obstructions. This means, first, begin the program of unpinching the existing pinched nerves—and you, like everyone else, have them. Secondly, eliminate the taking of drugs and gear your own body into manufacturing the drugs it can make and was created to make. Thirdly, don't further clog your plumbing with foodstuffs but eat only fruits for a week, giving the system a chance to rest itself and reorganize its forces and make itself well.

Chapter Twenty-Four

Building Up Your Heart

Are you a victim of, or scared to death by, heart disease?
Anyone in your family a victim?

Do you get nervous just thinking about coronary artery
disease, especially after hearing the alleged authorities hammering away at the statement that coronary occlusions are the nation's killer *numero uno?*

Take heart. We now can offer you known and tested ways
by which you may strengthen and induce repair processes in a
damaged heart.

We know exactly the kind of body movements that are
needed. What exercises to do—and when to do them—and *how
much* of any of them to do.

And we can tell you (as we do in the pages that follow) how
to assure an improved flow of nerve impulses, better called Life
Force, to the stricken heart by way of lead-in nerve pathways
from which the pressures or pinching blockages have been
removed.

You have heard me declare that a candle loses nothing by
lighting another candle. Better share what you are now about to
read with every adult of your acquaintance.

***

Exciting Research into Heart-Building Drills for Cardiacs

Everyone alive needs some exercise. Without activity of
some kind the body slows down, bones demineralize, metabolic

processes become sluggish and turgid. If only a daily walk of some distance, a walk with vigor and not just a slouching walk or leisurely stroll, daily exercise is needed.

Most of all, exercise is needed by the cardiac cripple. And he is the very one who is told to lie a-bed, take it easy, be super-careful about not exerting himself.

The exercise needed by the one who has had a heart attack is not the ordinary kind. He cannot, of course, run a race or play tennis or lift barbells. But with specific exercise tailored to his needs his heart will generally improve, not get worse.

The big thing for the cardiac is horizontal exercise. Never any exercise while sitting up or standing up. Any exertion or activity in the upright position forces the heart to accelerate immoderately while pumping blood *uphill*. To send blood to the upper chest, neck and head the heart overstrains because it has to lift the fluid in a straight uphill direction.

The great and beneficial exercise for heart attack victims is when they are lying down. Then the heart accelerates somewhat, of course, but this is good for it, as I will explain presently. What the heart does not do in the horizontal position is strain against gravity. It pumps blood to the lower extremities and abdomen—all organs *on the same level* with the heart, thus reached effortlessly. It pumps blood to the head and upper extremities, also *on the same level* and reached with relatively no effort.

Our experiments have revealed that tiny auxiliary blood vessels to the stricken portion of the heart tend to rebuild under a proper program of exercising the heart. As the *controlled activities* are continued, these little auxiliary arterioles feed into the stricken portion of the heart. This stricken portion is the part which does not receive its quota of blood because the coronary artery that is charged with doing this is occluded and cannot deliver. This is what is meant by coronary occlusion. But when the auxiliary little blood vessels serve that stricken portion of the heart with blood, the heart tends to mend unless it is irreversibly damaged—and most hearts I have found are not that far gone.

How to "Un-Damage" a Damaged Heart

What exactly are the *controlled activities* that tend to rebuild the damaged heart areas in this way? They are exercises done on the horizontal plane, exercises which I soon shall describe. They are all done lying down, preferably on a carpeted floor.

The best, I think, is the following: Lying on your back, raise the legs aloft and first wiggle the feet a bit. Look at the feet above you. Turn them in a circular and counter-circular movement, clockwise and counter-clockwise. The knees may be straightened out or bent a little, as you wish. Take your pulse. Learn to do this if you don't know how. Any nurses's aid can teach you. Say you find the pulse at around 70. Now bend the knees toward the chest alternately; bend each leg and straighten it aloft one after the other. It is like riding a bicycle upside down.

Do not fear that the pulse quickens. It should. You are flat on your back, solidly splinted against the floor and at rest. If you continue the alternate bending and straightening of your legs until your pulse reaches 100—not at all a dangerous level—those little auxiliary vessels to the heart that I spoke about will begin building and serving the area of the heart that is not receiving its proper blood supply from the occluded coronary.

I say this exercise is best because it can be performed moderately even by the very weak cardiac case. It is done within one's capacity to do. *Listen to the wisdom of the body.* While pedaling the imaginary bicycle aloft if your body says that only two or three revolutions of your legs are enough, that's it. Tomorrow your body will not tire before you do some four or five, and each day you will be able to increase the activity. But this is easy for anyone to do.

Another that vies with the foregoing as a "best exercise" is done on your hands and knees. Just take a step on your hands and knees, then another, then a third. Imagine yourself a four-footed animal. As such, your organs are in the right position for easiest, least exerting function. In a way this is even better than when lying on your back, for on your back the organs are forced to work upside-down as it were, pressed back and lying upon the backbone, while here they are forward and unhampered and able to perform best, without any construction.

Allow your head to hang downward, for this stretches the strong neck muscles—what doctors call the sternocleidomastoids—and tends to unpinch nerves in the neck. As you are on hands and knees with head hanging downward, traverse the length of your hallway if you can. Or walk around your living room. But do only as much as will give you a tired signal. When the body says you are somewhat, vaguely, even slightly tired, just stop. Quit for this day. Tomorrow you will be able to do more.

Now a third exercise that I have found to be a heart-rebuilding activity. This is also on hands and knees. Think now about the part of the backbone that people call the small of the back. Try to make this part of the back as hollow as you can. Dip it downward into as deep a hollow as possible. Having done this, arch it upward as high as you can. Now, as strength permits, go down and up, down and up, dipping and arching in succession. Just as soon as the tired signal appears, quit.

When I learned about these things I tried them on a group of cardiac sufferers with interesting results. At first I had only five in each test group. Five patients who had suffered heart attacks were permitted the conventional bed rest on the back and the inactivity that goes along with it. Five other cardiacs were given all three of the foregoing activities that I have denominated "best exercises" for heart victims. With only one well-remembered exception in those first early days of this research study, electrocardiographic tapes showed that the exercising patients improved. The improvement was both steady and regular. When the groups were later increased to 20 each, the results were even more clearly defined. With no exceptions at all those who exercised did better than the inactive cardiac patients.

I mentioned one well-remembered exception in my first

study. Upon inquiry I learned that the daily visits from this patient's wife were awesome affairs, for she nagged and irritated him almost to the point of inner explosion while innocently thinking she was being kind, and being considerate of his needs.

PUTTING IT ALL TOGETHER

If you have suffered a cornonary occlusion, or if you have had any kind of warning symptoms of an oncoming heart attack, or if you are worried because of a family tendency toward cardiac dysfunctions, these pages may be the most important you will ever read.

Do not just lie there and wait for the Grim Reaper. The body wants very much to be well. The body is self-healing, it forever tries to mend itself, to mend its damaged parts, just as you see your cuts and bruises mending all the time. The three exercises mentioned on pages 121 and 122 are designed to help and quicken the mending and heart-strengthening process.

Until you feel very strong, do not do any exercises in the conventional upright position. Do them all lying down.

Lie on your back and kick your legs around in circular fashion, as described above. When you have built up your pulse-beat from around 70 to 100 you may expect new auxiliary blood vessels to be developing for the purpose of serving any stricken portion of your heart, especially such portions not now properly served—because the coronary artery that is supposed to service it is occluded with sludge or plaques or some other toothpaste-like matter, which blocks the blood-flow through it.

Every morning, and especially before retiring every night, get on your hands and knees and "take a walk" around your house within your strength and capacity to do. Do not overtire. In a short while you will want to run a race on hands and knees.

Also on hands and knees, lower the small of the back into a deep hollow and raise it into a high arch. Do it slowly at first, later with as much vigor as strength will allow. Listen to the wisdom of the body.

Go Primordial

Much later, when strong and feeling energetic, try walking on hands and *feet,* not just on hands and knees. This is the one exercise that does "everything" for all parts of the body. When I discovered this "Primordial Walk" and first wrote about it in another book, more people indicated that they were helped by this one activity than by anything else I'd ever recommended. If you get to where you wish to do this Primordial Walk, please do it very carefully at first. Just a step or two is enough in the beginning.

A few more helpful items. Vitamin E has been shown to give enormous benefits to cardiac victims. Taking about 200 International Units after a meal—600 I.U.s daily—in my experience, has been an aid to every cardiac I've ever seen. In addition, a teaspoonful of powdered (debittered) yeast supplies the vitamin B that contains biotin, and biotin appears to be almost a specific for heart pains—all in the form of a natural food, not a drug at all. Also, I recommend one tablespoonful of lecithin granules plus one of cold-pressed soybean oil every day.

Oxygen, of course, is the real staff of life, and daily diaphragmatic breathing drills are recommended.

While on your hands and knees, head hanging down, open the lips slightly and pant like a dog, moving the mid-section in and out. This exercises the diaphragm, strengthens the breathing apparatus, and tends to reoxygenate the entire system. Do this especially at bedtime.

Also at bedtime, stand before an open window, or in the back yard or wherever the air is freshest, and fix your mind on those lower ribs of yours. Concentrating on them, spread them apart. Widen them. This opens the lower lobes of the lungs and enables you to store up a larger reservoir of life-giving air.

Before 10:00 and after 4:00, try to take a half hour of exposure to the sun on your bare body. Every day see that your bare feet are in contact with grass or earth—don't insulate yourself completely from Mother Earth and its emanations.

Eat small meals. Make them *very* small. Don't guzzle fluids of any kind. Sip, never swallow long draughts of any liquid. And do not permit saturated fats like lard or butter to enter your mouth. This goes, of course, for bacon and meat fats.

Note the toilet tissue after a bowel evacuation. If it is smeary, that's the test I've discovered that indicates improper or incomplete fat metabolism. Cut down your fat intake. When no hurtful fatty foods are entering your body you will discover that the toilet paper is relatively clean, never smeary.

Chapter Twenty-Five

Expanding Your Brain Power

The importance of this chapter lies in the fact that it gives you a rare secret, one that improves the memory and brain power—a secret employed by Aristotle, that most brilliant of many brilliant philosopher-scholars of ancient Greece.

If you believe that brain-power improvement and memory improvement are the result of long and expensive courses in mentalizing, mind control or whatever, you may be altogether wrong.

I dare you to try what I've written in the next page or two and not feel powerfully improved in both memory and thinking ability.

The best test to give this deliciously simple program is when you face a stiff examination or an ultra-important meeting with high-echelon people whom you very much want to impress. When you are going off to a conference where you will hammer out a contract that may affect your entire future— that's the time to try out what follows. When you are preparing a speech to deliver to an august body, and you are a bit nervous about speechmaking—give this method a try just an hour before your speech.

Ready? Well, let us all learn how to do what has hitherto been the secret of the gifted ones.
***

Dramatic Study of Aristotle and
Memory-Expanding Brain Power

Are you embarrassed by forgetfulness or faulty memory?

The enormously gifted Greek philosopher-scientist scholar, Aristotle, knew so much about so many things that he was called "Nature's private secretary."

One of the things he knew was how to make the brain cells pop: how to expand the mental horizons and make areas of the human brain function in bigger and better fashion than ever before. Aristotle knew how to awaken the brain and cause it to perform at the optimum level.

I have used the Aristotelian techniques both in my own life and with students in my classes who faced difficult examinations in anatomy, neurology and the like. I used to take, say ten students aside before a particularly difficult test that made them all apprehensive to the point of biting their nails. Before the examination I would put these ten through a half hour of Aristotle's magic brain exercises. The other students did not know of this and did not have the same preparation for the exams. The invariable results were almost amazing. The ten who *prepared their minds* with the Aristotelian drills were no longer afraid of the forthcoming examinations but actually anxious to sail into them. And they would finish the examinations before the others. Also, their marks generally were far above the average.

This proved to me that Aristotle's way of filling the mind with geometric figures and patterns in advance of *a heavy thinking event* was a kind of fodder for the mind and helpfully nourishing in the extreme.

In my own life, when preparing a study of involved and difficult elements, I used to do the drills I will now describe.

Make Lazy Brain Cells Pop into Activity

Close your eyes and imagine yourself standing in front of a blackboard. With an imaginery piece of chalk begin to draw a few geometric figures on the blackboard.

First draw a triangle on the board. Make it any size that is convenient. Around the triangle draw a circle. See in your mind that you now have before you a circle inside a square by drawing four sides around the circle.

Visualize what is before you on the blackboard. A square. Inside the square is a circle. Inside the circle you see a triangle.

Now place a cross on top of the three figures on the board. Make it a conventional cross, an equal-sided cross, any kind you like. Now that the cross is superimposed on the square, circle and triangle, superimpose a star over the cross. It may be a five-pointed, six-pointed or any other design you care to select. Now draw a rectangle or oblong on top of the star, placing it on the horizontal plane. After this draw in another oblong straight up and down on the vertical plane. Lastly, enclose all these figures within a large oval.

Eyes are still closed. You are visualizing what you have on that blackboard. An oval. Within the oval is a vertical oblong, under that a horizontal oblong, and under that a star. Under the star is a cross. If you should lift off the cross what you would have left are three figures: a square, circle, triangle.

Now, with eyes still closed, get rid of the figures you have drawn one by one. Begin with the last. Mentally, you reach up to the blackboard and take away the oval that encloses everthing. Throw the oval away. Now lift off and throw away the vertical oblong, then the horizontal oblong, then in turn the star, the cross, the square, the circle and the triangle.

In your mind "mock-up" two blackboards, one at each side of you about four feet apart and facing each other. You stand between the two blackboards with a piece of chalk in each hand. You can easily reach each blackboard with the chalk in each hand.

Now write the number 4 simultaneously on each board. Do this with left and right hands at the same time. Write the number 6 on each board. Now write 66, then 44, then 6644, then your own house number or telephone number or date of birth in numbers. Learn to write them at the same time on each side of you onto the blackboards facing you, between which you are standing. Being a mental drill, you are writing all these numbers in your imagination, not physically at all, and you can do it easily.

Try to see clearly the numbers you have written. In your imagination bring the two blackboards together; merge them into one. The numbers you have written now fit above each of their counterparts so that you have one set before you, just as though you had written them singly and not in pairs. Mentally eliminate the numbers one at a time, lift them off the blackboard and throw them away.

Continue with your eyes closed. Imagine yourself looking at yourself face to face. You see yourself in the mirror each day, but can you describe yourself? Suppose there were two of you. Suppose you were lost in the second person. Could you clearly describe you in the second person if asked by the police to do so?

Are you wide-eyed or are your eyes placed with only a narrow distance between them? Is your forehead high or low? Are your nostrils splayed wide and flaring or are they thin and delicate? Your chin: Is it square at the end, or thin and pointed, or rounded and uncreased? Are your lips very thin, and your mouth like a narrow line across your face? Are your lips thick? Rosebud shaped? Down-sloped into a frown? Up-curved into a humorous expression?

Get acquainted with the you that is you.

One more drill in this game that makes brain cells explode with unaccustomed activity. Imagine in detail the room in which you slept last night. With eyes closed see everything in that well-known bedroom of yours. See in your mind's eye the carpet, the color of the bedspread, the windows and curtains, if any. The chair, dresser, everything.

Now—note carefully. Imagine yourself sitting opposite your blackboard and on it you have a square, inside of which is a circle, inside of which is a triangle. While looking at the board and its geometric patterns before you, see this with only one eye, or with merely one side of your brain, while seeing your well-known bedroom with the other eye and other side of your brain. Try to see them both clearly, both at the same time. If you fail to see everything this first time, what is lacking now will become clear and in better focus on your next try.

Open your eyes. You have put yourself through an extraordinary mental drill. The gymnastics—all self-imposed while merely sitting in your chair—have made brain cells pop in your head that have never been used before.

Right now you are better prepared to tackle a difficult mental task than ever before. If you have really followed the foregoing experiment, you may at this moment discover that you have a quality you did not know you possessed. You can mentally write your name, or your friend's or spouse's name, on an imaginary blackboard and read the name both frontwards and backwards. The foregoing experiment and exercise makes the brain function at a higher level than before.

PUTTING IT ALL TOGETHER

You cannot *learn* any talent, of course, but you can develop whatever talent you were born with. You may never attain to the brilliance of an Einstein but you can develop the full potential of whatever skills and talents and genetic inheritance is yours.

The next time you are facing a difficult mental confrontation, do the foregoing drills. If you have to sign a contract and believe that the "party of the other part" may try to take advantage of you, prepare yourself with these gymnastics. If you must appear as a witness in court and need to be there with the clearest mind possible, go over these pages and do these blackboard workouts with geometric figures.

My publishers, all clever and knowledgeable people, will here learn for the first time that when I have a conference with them and want to be as alert as they are, I prepare for our editorial conferences with the Aristotelian drills.

Now the secret is out. Now they will do what I do and take away my advantage. Well, it was more important to me to share this with my readers than not to divulge it to my publishers!

Chapter Twenty-Six

Strengthening Your Breathing

In this polluted world many of us suffer from labored breathing, from asthma, from emphysema and associated syndromes.

Are you saddled with and victimized by breathing difficulties?

Because of the pollutants in the atmosphere there is very little we can do about *some* of this. But we can do a lot about *much* of this. There are ways by which we can "make do" with the poor quality of oxygen that the polluted atmosphere forces us to breathe into our lungs.

Dedicated ecologists on several fronts are mightily dedicated to the job of improving the world in which we live and breathe. But the power of commercial interests is very great. The various giant manufacturers may be expected to sicken our air and streams with industrial wastes, and we may as well expect to continue damaging our respiratory system every time we inhale air into our chests.

So—what to do?

Well, since there are areas about which we can do little or nothing, it becomes all the more important to improve our health in areas that we *can* do something about.

With all of this in mind I went into the research project recounted next, and I want you to know the story.

***

How to Strengthen the Breathing Apparatus

Since our atmosphere has become increasingly laden with pollutants, there has been an increase in emphysema and other "breathing diseases." We all hear the labored breathing of these victims on the streets, in theaters, trains, everywhere. Their coughing spells especially make one shudder.

Since it is breath and not bread that is the true staff of life, I have for many years been concerned with the breathing ability of my patients. Trying various ways to improve their breathing and oxygenating capacity, I finally settled on a few simple and workable items. My research efforts had paid off handsomely.

First, I had to settle for what I had to work with. We live in a polluted world. It was important to find a way whereby my people, those who paid me for advice and solid guidance of a meaningful *natural* sort, could learn to "make do" with the sadly existing air the best and most healthful way.

Secondly, I recalled what the wonderful Thoreau had said about being simple rather than complicated. What he urged was to "simplify, simplify, then simplify some more." The human body responds to simple techniques. Every truly helpful technique I had ever researched was in the end so embarrassingly simple that I wondered how it could have been missed for so many years.

Realizing that people with respiratory ailments needed to improve their breathing capacity, and that the environment was full of pollutants due to our substandard ecological conditions, I soon found how they could learn to "make do" with what poor oxygen was at hand. It was simply a matter of taking a few hundred international units of vitamin E every day. This has the near-magic property of allowing the organism to make out pretty well on a lower grade of oxygen. I finally settled on between 200 and 400 I. U.s of vitamin E daily, unless there was also a heart condition. With cardiac involvements I recommended 200 after each meal—600 International Units of vitamin E daily.

"Simplify, simplify, then simplify some more." With the vitamin E at hand I had the answer to how my emphysema and asthma people could live in a polluted world. With my chiropractic training I knew that they needed their existing nerves pressures corrected, so I devised self-help drills and techniques (given in Chapter Thirty-One) which instructed them how to unpinch their pinched nerves. Doing this, the nerve impulses to their poor breathing apparatus could reach the breathing muscles without interference, and the effect was like hooking into the electric outlet a machine that had not been plugged in. Without a normal flow of nerve impulses the breathing organs could not possibly work right, but now, with uninterrupted nerve-force flow through unpinched nerve pathways, the nerve pressure "unpinching drills" enabled the diaphragm and contiguous muscles to receive *life power* and work normally.

Count Twice as Long Exhaling As When Inhaling

But there still wanted one important factor. Since infancy most people were apical breathers. This means they breathed with only the apex of each lung, quite forgetting to use the big air-storage bins represented by the lower lobes of their lungs. Only the long distance runner, when he reaches what he calls "second wind," taps these enormous lung reserves or reservoirs of residual air. Thus, most people had weak breathing muscles and I had to search for ways to strengthen them—simple ways that they would follow, for I'd learned that my patients abhorred complicated instructions and seldom observed them.

At last I discovered an extraordinarily easy way to put those breathing muscles back to work full time and full capacity. The diaphragm had become semiparalyzed in most people from disuse, for they breathed with the apices of the lungs and did not use the diaphragm. If I strengthened the diaphragm back to normal power I'd get my people to draw air into the large lower lobes of the lungs and lick their respiratory problems. How could I achieve this? Why, just by tightening the diaphragm with every breath this main breathing organ would grow strong and powerful.

It was easy! Just tell them to count twice as long exhaling as they counted inhaling. Teach the people to get into the habit and rhythm of counting as they walked and breathed. As they took a breath *in,* they count to four or six, let's say. As they let the breath *out,* they count twice as long, rationing the breath out slowly to the count of eight or twelve.

Can you see what I was causing to happen? If they blew out the breath quickly it would only consume a count of one or two. To hold the breath to a count of twice what they counted inhaling it, they had to *parcel out the breath.* They had to let it out *under control.* Toward the end of their count the mid-section would tighten, the very powerful diaphragmatic muscle would be firming up, the entire breathing apparatus would be strengthening.

It was like a verifiable miracle. My patients who'd all their lives been shallow breathers or who'd had tendencies toward emphysema began to breathe like human beings. Their chests began to expand, their better intake and utilization of oxygen also gave them an unexpected gift of new-found happiness—that euphoria which flows from an inner sense of good health.

My patients were telling other people to count as they walked and breathed. It became a game. Some got to where they could measure their intake of air to the count of eight and ration the breath out slowly to the count of sixteen. Toward the end of the count the muscles in their mid-section would tighten like a clenched fist, and strengthen thereby. In the beautiful little city where I then practiced we developed a community of deep breathers.

Another technique for strengthening the human breathing apparatus proved equally simple—and, being uncomplicated, the patients followed it avidly. This was merely the business of raising the arms above the head, parting the lips slightly, and then panting like a dog. As one panted in this manner, the diaphragm (just below the breastbone) went in and out, in and out, in and out in unison. This is the chief breathing muscle of the body. As it went in and out it grew strong with the activity, it caused the lower lobes of the lungs to fill with a large storage reserve of air, it helped every aspect of metabolism because oxygenation is life in the best and truest sense.

PUTTING IT ALL TOGETHER

Beginning today, start up in your mind a kind of "gearing mechanism" that will cause you to do a counting routine while breathing. At first it will take conscious effort; then it will become automatic. Begin counting to four while you inhale. On exhaling, do it slowly in measured beats and count to eight. You will achieve a rhythm and enjoy the game. At night, just before retiring, stand before an open window or go into the yard or wherever the air is freshest, and raise your arms to pant like a dog with lips parted. Watch and enjoy the mid-section going in and out as the diaphragm moves. This will prepare you for a night of good sleep because it will oxygenate the entire system. Take a good brand of organic vitamin E daily, say between 200 and 400 International Units. Because it is a fat soluble, take the E vitamin after a meal—best after the meal at which you consumed the most fatty foods. Do the nerve-pressure unpinching drills given in Chapter Thirty-One of this book, and learn to count as you walk and breathe. Happy breathing!

Chapter Twenty-Seven

Reassessment of the
Mechanical Cause of Disease

Maybe neither drugs nor surgery are answers to what ails *you*. Perhaps *your* ailment was originally caused by a mechanical upset: a jarring impact or fall that moved mechanical parts of the body out of position, and pressed on nerves or threw organs out of mechanical alignment, and made it impossible for the organs to do the job for which they were intended. Then you'd need mechanical attention by a doctor trained in bodily mechanics.

In such case no drug or injection could possibly normalize a mechanically caused fault—an ailment or upset such as a curvature, a vertebral displacement, a subluxation (as they are called) which results in nerve pressure, a low shoulder, a high hip, a short leg, a neck which cannot be turned equally in both directions, et cetera.

As I have written elsewhere—and something that needs repeating and repeating— the human body is not only a chemical factory but also a machine. It is a machine with moving parts in it. Those moving parts are subject to being strained or jarred out of position, especially the way we live against gravity and sustain strains and stresses in our daily workaday lives. And when any part of the body gets out of alignment the entire body is out of adjustment.

Better read on.

***

Dramatic Reassessment:
The Chemical Vs. Mechanical Cause of Disease

Everyone alive is concerned about his sickness and health. In every crowd and on every train or bus one can hear conversations about what this doctor said, the other doctor did and third doctor was going to do.

Always, it appears, this is in some way related to medicines. The medicine one takes and needs to take. The drugs that are being elaborated or researched to reach human illnesses. The brilliant progress of modern medical science.

Have you ever considered that all this goes at the business of human health by only one route? It approaches health and disease through only one door—the chemical door.

Whenever you are discussing medicines or drugs you are talking about the chemical way to health. It relates to what doctors call the *chemical cause* of disease.

Why do not doctors in general open *all* the doors that lead to all known causes of human disease? One would think that all disease is chemically caused. Much of it, however—and some say most of it—is mechanically caused, and for this there are no drugs at all.

From the concentration on drugs and medicines, all of which are chemical, and from all the conversation about drug-prescribing doctors and hospitals that go at human disease chemically, one would hardly guess that there exists the almost universal, very widespread cause of disease that is purely mechanical and not chemical at all.

Reducing it down to essentials, it may be said with validity that there are two major causes of disease in the world. They are the chemical cause and the mechanical cause. The body goes awry chemically, in most cases, *after* it goes askew mechanically. *To save your life this must be understood.*

It is known—and known very well by scientists—that the human body makes its own drugs. The body manufactures all the adrenalin and cortisone and insulin it needs for its health and its growth and its self-repair. It has the capacity to manufacture all its needed pepsin and hydrochloric acid and hormones and enzymes merely out of the food one eats, the fluids one drinks and the air one breathes.

If the body has this capacity—why did it stop using it? Why did the body quit manufacturing its needed cortisone or HCl? Did the body just capriciously—merely impulsively—decide to quit manufacturing the insulin and adrenalin and pepsin it needs? Or—note well—did *something* happen to cause it to quit doing and manufacturing what it was set up to do and make?

What could that *something* have been?

Is Your Ailment Mechanically or Chemically Caused?

Well, consider this fairly and objectively. We live in defiance of gravity. We are not solidly posted on four legs in the manner of the horizontal, four-legged animal. Living and heaving and lugging and tugging in a straight up-and-down contra-gravity position, we twist and fall and strain and suffer daily mechanical impacts which cause our bodily parts to get worked or strained out of position. When this happens the vertebral bones of our spinal column, for example, pinch nerves. If such nerves are charged with conveying functional impulses to the stomach, it can follow that the peptic and pyloric glands in the stomach quit manufacturing natural pepsin. If there are pinched nerves serving the pancreas, the pancreas is then deprived of the energizing impulses it needs and this may cause it to stop secreting and elaborating and manufacturing insulin. And so it goes. This is *that something* that may be the cause of most human disease. This is precisely what may be holding up our ability to gain over cancer, heart disease, diabetes, arthritis and other rising rather than diminishing degenerative diseases.

Now there remains but one important point to cover. In any restudy of the chemical cause of disease as opposed to or contrasted with the mechanical cause, the big question to ask is this: Is human disease more likely to be caused chemically or mechanically? That is the question. If an imbalanced body chemistry causes diseases most often, then clearly the chemical approach should be employed more often. If disease is most often caused by structural mechanical upsets of the body, then drug approaches should be forsworn and mechanical treatments should be offered to the sick who are crying to get well.

Very well. Let us view the matter with scientific knowledge and relentless logic. We know that we can pinch off a nerve that serves power to the stomach and the result will be a diminution or complete cessation of pepsin and/or hydrochloric acid manufactured there. This is a chemical ailment for which pepsin or store-bought HCl is prescribed—*a chemical ailment caused by a mechanical pressure on nerves.* Similarly, a mechanical strain or fall can cause a shift in a vertebra and mechanical pressure on nerves to the supra-renal glands, gall bladder or wherever, with a resulting chemical upset or ailment in the common bile duct or in such diseases as hypoadrenia.

We know of no way by which a chemical imbalance, coming first, can in turn cause a mechanical upset, however. The human body can get strained out of mechanical whack and cause a disease of a chemical nature. A disease of a chemical nature cannot, however, cause the human body to get out of mechanical whack!

After more than forty years as a researching and dedicated doctor of the mechanical school of healing, but one who also knows the chemical approach to human disease, I am convinced that most ailments are precipitated by mechanical upsets in the body. I know that in our daily style of contra-gravity living there is more opportunity for straining ourselves out of balance *mechanically* than getting out of balance *chemically*. And I know that in my long career I have personally, at times, accomplished the correction of almost every known ailment *by mechanical treatments alone,* often in cases that came to me for help after being told by medical (chemical) doctors that nothing could be done for them.

I believe firmly and almost unalterably that a great change for good would ensue if merely one thing were done in our hospitals. I refer to a change that would require every patient referred to major surgery to be first also seen by a doctor of my kind who would examine such patient for mechanical causes of the existing trouble, upon finding which, of course, the mechanical correction would be made if at all reversible. If this one thing were done I am convinced there would be far fewer surgeries performed, and far greater numbers would leave hospitals with good natural health and less hospital time required.

I am convinced beyond peradventure of a doubt that if all sick persons were examined for both chemical causes and mechanical causes, it would be discovered that a staggeringly greater number are sick because of mechanical rather than chemical reasons.

PUTTING IT ALL TOGETHER

You were born with a complete chemical factory but not with complete mechanical equipment. At birth your hundred organs could already perform a thousand functions, all with precision and without confusion, manufacturing all the chemical drugs (insulin, pepsin, hydrochloric acid, hormones, adrenalin) you need, and manufacturing all this out of the food and fluid you consumed plus the air you breathed. *But at birth you could not even sit up* because your mechanical equipment was not yet complete. Later you taught yourself to live in defiance of gravity. You urged yourself, and adapted your body, to stand, balance, walk, run, heave, lug, tug, strain, twist, turn, hit chuck holes that jarred your spine, take mis-steps and jolts to your mechanical structures. This pushed or bounced or strained bodily parts out of normal proper position, pinching blood vessels and especially blocking nerves. When nerves became blocked (as we find that some *are* blocked in almost everyone) they interfered with the conductivity of functional life power to organs. Then the deprived organs got sick—all because of mechanical cause, and were no longer able to manufacture the needed chemical ingredients they were created to manufacture.

All this means one great thing for you and your health. If ailing in almost any way whatever, first see to it that your body is mechanically in order, not malpositioned. Without the body's being in proper mechanical shape it cannot reasonably be expected to perform the jobs it was intended to do. If lacking in hydrochloric acid, for example, do not take drugstore HCl, but *first* do some of the drills in Chapter Twelve to readjust, or un-pinch, any nerves to the stomach that may be pinched, and probably are. If you cannot quite make it by yourself, or if it is a dire emergency, get a chiropractic doctor to do it for you as a starter, then carry on entirely on your own. Once the nerves to the stomach are unblocked of pressure, they will deliver *Life Power* to the stomach, the stomach will be able with this renewed functional power to again manufacture the needed stomach digestive acid, and you will have gained and main-tained health by yourself—by avoiding the doctors.

Here are some final words to remember on this most im-portant subject. It is a subject which, if understood, will forever serve as your Primer for Protection.

Your organism, as indicated, is not only a chemical factory but also a machine. It is a mechanical contrivance. It is a machine made up of many movable parts. No machine with moving parts in it can operate 24 hours a day as your body does for years on end and fail to get out of adjustment or mechanical balance. And no machine that is out of adjustment can be *reasonably* expected to work properly or function normally.

The human being gets out of mechanical adjustment far more often than he gets out of chemical balance. Note one shoulder lower than the other, so low that the tailor has to insert a shoulder pad to make you appear even. Note that one earlobe is lower than the other, one shoulderblade sticks out farther than its mate, one leg may be shorter than its opposite number, your chin may not be exactly under your nose but off to one side of it.

The 2-Scale Test

Stand on two bathroom scales with your feet equidistantly apart and note that you may weigh ten or more pounds heavier on one side when you should be exactly the same if you are in mechanical balance. Note how you always cross your knees in one favorite direction, recrossing occasionally only for a moment's rest but going back to the favorite side quickly, and ask a chiropractic doctor what this denotes with respect to the malposition propensities of your lower spine. Stand before an ordinary string or plumbline suspended from the ceiling and note how it does not bisect you square in the middle of your body as it should but usually trails off to one side or the other, showing how far offside and off balance you are mechanically.

Remember that when the body is out of mechanical alignment it can *cause* the body chemistry to get out of balance, for any nerve pressures may prevent or curtail an organ's ability to manufacture its needed enzymes or secretions. But you may be sure that mere chemical imbalance cannot cause any such mechanical fault in the body as a nerve-root compression. Thus, mechanical faults should be attended to *first*. Yet medical men hardly ever even examine the spine, which is the central nerve panel and switchboard of the body, much less know what to do about nerve pressures if they found any.

Read well what is herein written. Go to the last chapters and read well and heed well. Then, barring the most grave cases, you will be your own doctor.

Chapter Twenty-Eight

Freeing Yourself from Pinched Nerves

Do you have a problem with cervical nerve pressure, or pinched nerves in the neck?

If your problem has been a wry neck (or torticollis) you may have noticed that the condition seemed to come and go; in other words, you've probably had a succession of attacks of this pesky condition.

This is beyond a doubt due to a weakness in the nerve-distribution pattern in your neck, and I have discovered an effective manner of dealing with it. It can be done at home, almost always by yourself, without the help of any other person whatever.

If you think it foolhardy to try to make a diagnostic neck test on yourself, have another think, please. The method outlined for you here is utterly simple.

Moreover, I consider that the techniques given here for the correction of nerve pressures in the neck—corrections that you can make all by yourself—are really beyond price in most cases.

***

The Technique of Determining and Correcting One's Own Nerve Pressures in the Neck

I can recall a time in my researching career when I felt that most human ailments were caused by, or at least contributed to by, nerve pressures in the neck.

As the years went by I became even more certain of this. Twenty years after the original thought-wave hit me, I knew more than ever that the human neck gets out of trouble, and presses upon nerves, and causes ailments more often than any other one area of the body. The original thought was a kind of pre-vision. It turned out to be verifiable perspicacity.

Now I can explain it all. I can tell the reader how to measure *for himself or herself* whether he or she has nerve pressures anywhere in the neck. And I can tell you how to make the correction. Make it at home. Make it all by yourself, without any doctor needed at all. Only in rare cases, or exceedingly grave ones, will it be necessary to enlist professional help, and in such cases my firm opinion is that the professional ought to be a chiropractic doctor.

First, there is one thing you must understand about the neck. It has a number of muscles that can pull it from side to side and work the head in all directions. Two muscles are especially heavy and strong, and they can shorten or get into a spasm and yank the head off to one side into what is called a wry neck or torticollis condition. Occasionally I hear orthopedic surgeons refer to these powerful neck muscles as "those SCM factors"—SCM meaning sternocleidomastoid, which is the name for these muscles—but in all my years of contact with ordinary medical men in general practice I have never known one to refer to these great protective muscles of the neck or even so much as glean their importance.

Now, about that neck of yours. In the case of a four-legged animal that spends its life in a horizontal position, these powerful SCM muscles are elongated because the animal's head is down as it grazes. Being stretched, relaxed, elongated to full length, these muscles rarely get into trouble and rarely squeeze or pinch any nerves, blood vessels, transmitting pathways of any kind. But—now note this. Since man stood up on his hind legs and became a walking two-legged person, the neck is no longer elongated but *curved.* It curves inwardly *into a hollow* and the head is precariously balanced on top of this curved neck, held in delicate position by neck muscles, mostly by these SCM powerhouse muscles.

In this position you often sustain what you inelegantly call a "crick in the neck." You turn suddenly in answer to a call.

You wheel round at a sound of danger. You wiggle taking a dress off over the head. A cold draft hits the neck on one side during sleep while the other side is snug against the warm pillow. The sternocleidomastoid shortens, it pulls the head to one side while the chin points in the opposite direction. You have a stiff neck, a "crick," a condition professionally labeled torticollis.

What you have is pressure on nerves. You suffer from nerve-root compression, with all kinds and manners of symptoms and ailments possible as a result. Or you have a simple neck immobility that may be easily corrected before any deep and grave maladies stem from it.

Now, please, get this! *Half the people in this world have pinched nerves in their neck to some degree,* in my carefully studied opinion. Half the people *everywhere* walk around with cervical nerve pressures, and with symptoms caused by such nerve pressures, AND ARE BEING TREATED FOR EVERYTHING IMAGINABLE EXCEPT THESE CAUSATIVE NERVE PRESSURES.

How do I know this? How can I make you know this, too? Easy. The technique follows.

Since half of all human beings, especially adults, suffer from pinched nerves in the neck, how can we tell which half? Half the four billion people on this planet, I am sure, have this condition of neck-nerve pressures—half the people who read this book have it, half of the people in your family have it. So you want to know which half—or who—or if it also applies to *you*.

Give Yourself a Spinal Adjustment

All right. Stand in front of a mirror, facing it straight front. Turn your head as far to the right as you can. Out of the corner of your eye note the distance between your chin and the tip of your shoulder. Is the tip of your chin two inches from the shoulder tip, or three inches, or more, or less? Note it. Now turn the head as far to the left as you can do *naturally,* without straining. Does it turn the same distance—or just as far—to the left as it did toward the right?

This is the determinant. Here you have your measuring gauge. If you have *unequal* mobility of the neck you do have nerve pressure in the neck. This is a certainty, a well-researched mechanical fact of the body, not a guess.

Let's put it another way. If you cannot turn your neck as far one way as the other way, you have a shortening of neck muscles and pinched nerve routes in your neck. In that case there may be sickness in the organ that is served by the pinched nerves, because the nerve impulses needed by the organ for its work aren't getting through the pinched nerve in proper force, quality or quantity. If the organ served by such a pinched nerve is not sick, then it must be on the way to becoming sick because it is *deprived* of the nerve impulses it requires for its daily function, coordination, operational direction.

If this sounds bad, it is bad only if neglected.

The good news is that these unequal neck mobilities can be corrected. The technique is quite easy, as you will soon see. The difficult part was to research it out, find it, recognize it. Once recognized, we know what's there and know what to do about it.

Here is what to do.

Facing the mirror, bring your arms up and bend them so that the elbows are pointing toward the mirror. This places your hands alongside your neck. Cup your neck in the palms and fingers of your hands, the fingers partly gripping the back of the neck. Do not press inwardly to choke yourself but hook under those projecting bones (mastoid portions) and *lift straight up.* Lift as hard as you can in a straight upward direction. Do it with the head tipped forward a little, not bent back into a neck hollow.

Just gripping the neck like this and lifting upward in a straight line (with the head tipped forward a bit) will help all by itself. The only thing to watch is that your hands at the sides of the neck don't press toward center to choke off your breathing but expend their effort in an upward and slightly forward direction.

Now, the real nub or gist of this technique. As you lift, also turn your head as far right as you can, then while still lifting turn as far left as you can.

Do not slacken your upward lift as you turn the head. The tendency will be to forget to lift as you think about turning the head. Lift and turn. Turn as far as you can in both directions.

Now, as a sophisticated piece of doctoring technique, try this: Note which direction you were able to turn the head *farther* in the test before you began the lift business. Let us say it was the right. You were able to turn the chin closer to the right shoulder than to the left when you tested for neck mobility. Very well, now lift as directed and turn the head even farther toward the right. You may neglect the side that was short. Concentrate on the side where you could already turn farther, and lift it while you turn it even farther. I know it doesn't sound right to you, but that's because you have not studied and researched the cross pull of the muscles here. Just try it as I say. Lift and turn the head toward where you already could turn the head farther, then discover with a thrill that the other side, where you were short, has evened out. Or it has come more nearly even.

To the extent that you have lengthened the distance of head-turning by this technique, you have diminished or eliminated nerve pressures in your neck.

If you have problems of tinnitus, or are hard-of-hearing, note what happens after these neck lifting and neck-turning drills. Note the diminution of head noises, whistling or drumming or roaring in the ears; and note how your hearing capacity increases, with less tension and nerve strain to hear what is said around you.

I have instructed even epilepsy cases with grand mal-seizures to do this, and just this technique alone has in several cases reduced not only the frequency but also the severity of the seizures. I can recall one case several years ago where, in enthusiasm, the young lady stopped taking her bromides and dilantin altogether, all in one sweep, and still had fewer and less severe attacks than heretofore—all because she did this one drill several times a day.

Of one thing you may be sure, that this technique can only help and *cannot do injury* except, possibly, in cases of Pott's disease (tuberculosis of spine) which is rare indeed. But in spinal bone tuberculosis the disease is already known and the person is already braced. Even then, if done lightly, there is much possible good to be derived from this lift-and-turn neck mobility-equalizing technique, for it opens the life-giving nerve supply and enhances healing processes.

PUTTING IT ALL TOGETHER

Since the downflow of nerve impulses from the spinal cord through the neck can affect any condition to which man is heir, do this no matter what ails you. Just try it in front of a mirror. Turn the head both ways and note if you can turn equally far in both directions. If not, then in my view it is impossible for you *not to have* some nerve pressure in the neck. Raise your elbows, bring open hands backward against the sides of your neck, hook under the protruding mastoid processes and lift. Don't resist the lift, don't do this by curving the head backward, but lift upward and even a bit forward. This means your head will be an inch or two forward of straight up. Lift and turn. Lift and turn especially in the direction where you can turn *farther*. This sounds odd to you, for you will want to lengthen the short side, but do it as here directed.

Last thing at night, when in bed and flat on your back, take the neck tensions and nerve compressions out from the day's straining activities. Reach your open hands back and cup the sides of the neck between them. Lift straight back toward the headboard of the bed and turn the head meanwhile. Turn especially, or altogether if you wish, toward the side where you can turn farther. Then, on rising, note how much your neck mobility has improved. Tell others to do it and see them benefit.

Chapter Twenty-Nine

Improving Weak Eyes

In this little chapter I address myself to those who have weak eyes.

Also to those whose eyes tire easily. Eyes that burn or itch or water a lot. Eyes, moreover, that are far too sensitive to ordinary sunlight.

All persons who wear glasses ought to acquaint themselves with the information and techniques that the following research project produced. Some of this is incredible. All of it is greatly beneficial and beyond what the conventional eye people with conventional eyeglass prescriptions have achieved.

So read well what appears in the following pages, those of you with astigmatic problems, with nearsightedness and farsightedness, with inadequacy or uncoordination of the eye muscles, certainly those who have apparently irremediable headaches (migraines) referable to the eyes.

With so many millions in our land suffering eye difficulties or needing the support of crutches named eyeglasses, this may be exactly what you have been wanting to know.

***

Some Easy, Natural Ways to Improve the Eyes

The occulists and optometric people estimate that there are 93 millions in the United States of America who wear glasses.

When I began researching this field I went back to first principles. Where did we begin to go wrong? At once the answer springs to mind. Man was made to rise at sun-up and retire at sunset, using his eyes only while there was light from above. Man went wrong when he began living a large part of his life in the dark evening hours under artificial light, thus punishing his eyes as they were never intended to be punished.

About this there is little we can do. Certainly we are not about to give up our lifestyle and cut out living after dark. So, although it is nice to see our fault from the original stem, we must come to grips with the realities and conclude that we will not be able to do anything for human eyesight in this quarter.

But in addition to abusing and punishing human eyes under artificial electric light, there is another huge and unexplored area of *eye-hurtingness* about which we can do something.

Please think this through with me.

How We Use Our Eyes Incorrectly

We do all our reading with eyes glued straight in front of us, unwaveringly looking at the book held before the face. We watch television by the hour with eyes straight front. I am sitting and typing this page with eyes straight front. You do your sewing, driving, everything with eyesight employed in only one rigid direction—straight front.

The human eyeball is almost spherical in shape. It has muscles attached to it that work it forward and sideways. When you strain *straight frontward,* the muscles of front vision are working and pulling and activitating the eye in a forward direction. But the muscles of side vision are inactive, not employed, giving all the play on the eyeball to the front muscles. So what do you suppose happens?

The eyeballs are pulled *out of round.* The front muscles *overwork* because we do all our reading, sewing, driving and such in a straight front direction. The muscles of peripheral vision, which are the side muscles, *underwork* because, unlike the animals that see in a full 180-degree arc, we rarely look sideways. Thus the overworking and overpulling front muscles elongate the eyeballs. From front to back the eyeballs are no longer spherical. The light, as it enters the eyes, no longer converges at the same place where it would if the eyeballs were not elongated. So you cannot see so well, and the eye doctor has lenses ground to shape them in such a way that the entering light does hit the retina at the right point. Then you see again properly. But only with the help of eye-crutches.

I have tried to make the above clear. If you do not quite follow it, reread the previous paragraph until you do. Then all that flows and follows from this point onward will be clear to you.

If you begin to do the drills and exercises that I will set forth in these pages presently, one thing will start to happen for sure. By doing the exercises that use your muscles of side vision, those very muscles will get strong. They will begin to pull on your eyeballs sideways. They will tend to pull your eyeballs away from the elongated shape back into spherical shape.

Then you may begin to notice a curious thing. Although the glasses you wear may be newly fitted, your eyes may now bother you and your vision may become uncomfortable. You go back to the eye doctor and are told a strange thing. "I don't understand it," he may say. "These glasses are relatively new, but something has happened and you need others. These are for some reason too strong for you. You need *less correction* now than you needed just a few months ago."

Almost everyone can begin to reshape his eyeballs, regardless of age. By the drills which follow, the eyeballs will tend to get back into round from their out-of-round shape. Now that you will be inclined to follow what is here set forth. In my doctoring years I have learned that by sharing all explanations with the patient I get a participating patient, the very best kind. They don't like to be treated as though they are too stupid to understand what the doctor is doing, and why. If the doctor will but take the time to include them in all his work on their problems, and explain all sides of the work to them, they would be delighted and more cooperative because it then becomes a joint effort, a partnership. My own finding has been that very often the doctor does not explain too fully because alas, he does not himself understand it too fully.

PUTTING IT ALL TOGETHER

Prepare to "think sideways" and make use of your muscles of side vision in a few new and remarkably helpful, corrective ways.

First, when riding in a car as a passenger (not driver), hold a card in front of your eyes to shut out central vision. Out of the sides of your eyes you will be able to see the passing cars, telephone poles, buildings. You will be using peripheral muscles only, those that work to pull your eyeballs sideways.

In the glove compartment of most cars are folded maps or cards you can always employ for this technique. Merely hold it on the nose so that you cannot see frontward, thus forcing yourself to use side vision. After a few minutes of watching the passing objects through the sides of your eyes, do not be surprised to find yourself tired. The eyes, being unaccustomed to peripheral vision, will signal fatigue. When this happens, the following is the technique for resting and rejuvenating the organs.

Squeeze the eyelids together very tightly, then open them and flutter or blink them rapidly. Squeeze and flutter several times in succession. When you squeeze the lids tightly you force blood out of the capillaries or tiny arteries. When you open the lids and flutter them, new fresh blood nutrition flows in. By repeating these squeezes and flutterings you are starting a beneficial "pumping action" to the strained, weak, overworked eyes.

Now do the three things that most human eyes fall short of doing, and suffer thereby. *One:* Roll your eyes within closed sockets. See a large clock in you mind and roll the eyes from 12 o'clock on top clockwise around to the same spot, then counterclockwise, doing this until a little tired. *Two:* Bathe your eyes in their own lubricating fluid by working the eyeballs form side to side and up and down, and also in diagonal movement, to give them a full workout. *Three:* Hold the forefingers of both hands in front of your face, eyes open, and extend the fingers sideways while following them with your eyes. To be sure you see each finger out of the corner of each eye, wiggle the fingers. Besides doing this sideways, extend the fingers, and bring them to center, then extend them again on a diagonal plane.

Sit between two persons, look at them, close your eyes and "think sideways." See them in your mind's eye. Actually roll your eyeballs sideways in their closed sockets, lubricating them again in their own fluid, and see the people, walls, objects on each side of you. This practice strengthens the muscles of side vision and inclines to re-shaping the out-of-round eyeballs.

Just the above drills of holding a card before the eyes, plus the three immediately preceding, merely these have so improved eyesight problems in my research groups that glasses have been discarded after many years of needing them. Also, unbelievably enough, some difficult cases of migraine headache not amenable to other forms of treatment have been entirely cured. These were cases referable to eye difficulties, the migraines coming as the result of untreated or improperly treated visual problems.

If you have dark sunglasses, discard them except for use when driving directly into the sun when nonuse would be dangerous. Arthritic persons have been known to improve when discarding their dark lenses, for photosynthesis and vitamin D conversion takes place through the eyes to a large extent, a matter not possible when sunglasses are used.

It is important to learn not to stare. Learn to see an object wholly, not stare at a pinpoint. If you look at a finger, for example, see the skin, the knuckles, the nail and all, all at the same time, but don't stare at any one wrinkle in the skin. To stare is to hurt human vision. Learn to *see without looking*. This is something to learn. Think of the lens of a camera. It makes no effort to see; it only sees what flows into its line of vision. Try to think of a camera lens and use your eyes similarly.

Chapter Thirty

Diets for All Seasons and Conditions

The Diet for Losing Weight Naturally and Effectively

The trouble with losing weight by dieting, or by fasting, is that the weight is put back on as soon as one starts eating or quits dieting.

We all know people who have lost weight by way of erratic crash diets, by way-out harmful programs, and even by disciplined noneating fasting schedules, only to have put it all on, and sometimes even more, when the effort was completed and normal or former eating habits were resumed.

This doesn't have to be so. I myself have directed eating programs, and also plenty of fasts, where the patients held what weight they'd won, or held it close to their desired weight, depending on what the temptations of their social life were and what self-discipline they used in not stuffing themselves with unneeded food items.

In my career I have learned some strange and almost unbelievable things about dieting and the effects of dieting. One is that you can lose weight on almost any kind of diet. The other is that you seemingly can improve your health *for a time* on almost any kind of diet.

Do you know that you can lose weight not only by fasting or by a restricted, 1,000-per-day-calorie diet, but also by consuming hardly anything more than fatty food items? The body appears to resent such lopsided programs and sheds weight (meanwhile also shedding health) until you stoke its inner furnace with properly balanced nutrients. One doesn't feed milk into a gasoline tank or water into an oil-burning receptacle. One cannot give the human body a noncarbohydrate program where even fruits and vegetables are eliminated, or virtually an all-protein regiment where the plumbing piles up vast stores of harmful putrefactive acids, and come away from it all unscathed. One loses weight all right, but at what cost? None of us wants a weight loss at the expense of destroying the rhythm of metabolic processes or hammering on the neurological workings of the organism.

Just the same, no matter how odd and one-sided the eating program may be, for a while one appears to feel better. Why is this so? I am sure that this happens because the body is rested in this manner from the usual pilings-on of slop and *unfoods* that constitute the usual eating programs of most people. If you have nothing but grapefruits seasoned with lemon juice for reducing, or nothing but meat and lettuce, or even bacon and butter and mayonnaise, the body will at least be rested from having thrown into it such an awful variety of indigestibles and uncombinables at single meals that it feels better just because of the vacation from usual abuses. But this is only for a time. Then the liver acts up, the plumbing gets clogged, even muscle areas show unexpected weakness to the point where the smallest exertions result in hernias.

There exists a perfect way to lose weight and hold the weight down. Several ways, in fact. All of them work admirably. One is my favorite because it keeps everyone comfortable and happy.

Plan One

Fast for up to seven days. Almost everyone except a TERMINAL CANCER CASE or at times a serious CASE OF NEPHRITIS, can do this with profit. If in doubt, go to a doctor and have yourself checked beforehand. Do not be very active during this week of fasting. Sip, never guzzle, just as much water as you need to satisfy real thirst, but do not drink just to be drinking.

After seven days, take orange juice or tomato juice diluted

with water, half of each, in small two-ounce sips every two hours. If you desire you may have diluted orange juice at one period and tomato juice (from fresh tomatoes) as an alternate. That is all for the first day.

On the second day have small sips of carrot juice plus steamed zucchini squash. This is the most tender of vegetables, I have found, and irritates no intestinal lining even after a most rigid fast. No seasoning whatever, eat very small portions, masticate each mouthful a long time, and after a noneating schedule of a week this squash will taste like authentic heaven.

After two such days of preparation for eating following the one-week fast, go for a full week on the MONO-DIET as given in the following section. Thereafter keep the protein intake down to no more than two ounces daily, which is about what one finds in eight ounces of cheese or wheat germ or sunflower seeds. And satisfy yourself between meals with small sips of buttermilk. And take a multivitamin-multimineral tablet once a day.

The trick here, if trick it be, is the buttermilk. Sip at all day long if you want. It will keep the stomach happy, your innards not craving anything, and your weight down. This is my most comfortable weight-losing plan. Fast for a week, do not quaff water but sip it, follow with dilute juices for a day and combined carrot juice and zucchini for another day, then the Mono-Diet program, which is almost "perfection perfected" for what you seek, and after a week of this eat small portions of protein, frequent sips of buttermilk, and a daily supplement of vitamins and minerals. Following the week on the Mono-Diet, raw salad plates without salt may be had as often as desired.

Plan Two

No fasting at all. Only a way of keeping the inner stomach walls happy by giving them a sense of fullness and always something to work on.

Cut up a head of cabbage into quarters and eat a quarter of a cabbage head right out of your hand whenever you feel hungry. Do this with lettuce also if you like. No seasoning at all, unless you wish to squeeze a bit of lemon juice over it. Try to masticate the raw cabbage or lettuce so thoroughly that your own saliva will supply the fluids you need. Keep fluid intake down—almost nothing. Between meals of raw cabbage or lettuce, take small sips of buttermilk, only drop by drop, as often as you like all day long. This keeps the stomach full, you don't even know you are dieting, and the weight loss is great.

In masticating the raw cabbage or lettuce, count as many as 30 chews before swallowing each mouthful. After a week of this, which usually results in a huge weight loss, take one day on diluted juices and one day on juices plus steamed zucchini squash as in Plan One, then the Mono-Diet which wonderfully *stabilizes your weight* and holds it where it should be. The rules of low protein intake, very small fluid intake, and daily mineral-vitamin supplementation also apply here. One sure way to keep yourself from returning to former obese proportions is this: Never take any fluids such as soup, coffee, tea, soda, juice, water *unless it is in answer to a real thirst signal* coming out of your body and demanding that thirst be quenched. Just to drink in answer to the social "What are you drinking today?" habit is a sure way to balloon your body with wrong fluid weight all over again.

Plan Three

Three full days on watermelon only. Cut the fruit into small pieces of perhaps one ounce each. Eat one such piece about every hour during the day. It is more like taking a drink than having food. Be prepared to urinate a great deal, for this is a powerful natural diuretic. Take no other food or fluid at all. After three days go on as many raw salad plates as you care to consume, seasoned only with lemon juice, plus a small dish of raw wheat germ with skimmed milk daily. Follow this for as long as a full week. Then the very helpful Mono-Diet plan for a week or two, taking vitamin-mineral supplements daily, and after that a regular low-protein regimen of small meals, very low fluid intake, and frequent sips of buttermilk to keep the insides happy while the body firms and the weight stays down.

***

The Diet for Strengthening a Weak Heart

In most cases when we speak of a weak heart we refer to coronary artery disease. This is the condition where one of the two coronary arteries that lead to the heart (sometimes counted as three because of the branching), are occluded or blocked. When this happens the heart does not receive the blood it needs for its work. The portion of the heart thus deprived of needed blood cries with sharp pain from its stricken state. Somehow we must find a way to get rid of the plaques and other "sludge" which collects on the inside of the coronary like toothpaste.

There are other conditions that make one's heart "a weak heart" in layman's parlance. There are inflammatory conditions of the inner or outer linings of the heart or of the heart muscle itself, there are problems with the valves of the organ and a variety of other kinds and types of dysfunction. But, really, it hardly matters because the wonder of *natural healing techniques* is that they tend to heal the sick heart no matter whether the diagnostic label happens to be infarction, fibrillation or any of the things mentioned above. The body just *absolutely wants to get well* if given half a chance, for the human organism tends toward the normal (as when you cut a finger and it proceeds to heal at once, without a diagnosis), and through the plan set forth in this volume you do indeed give the ailing heart more than half a chance.

On the *level of diet* our plan is to *naturally* try to get rid of the sludge in the plugged heart arteries, get the arteries to *naturally* dilate, normalize and balance the blood chemistry so that there is no functional or metabolic strain forced upon the heart.

Coupling this with the other advice on the *level of regular and moderate exercise,* the kind that is right for the cardiac sufferer and within his capability to do and with our drills to remove nerve pressures on pathways to the heart, the cardiac patient has the best chance in the world to get well if his condition is at all reversible, which most are.

The proper exercises for the cardiac, those which tend to

build in tiny auxiliary vessels to the stricken portion of the heart in coronary occlusion—such exercises have been given earlier in this book and will be repeated in Chapter Thirty-One.

The techniques for unpinching pinched nerves to the heart—these have also been set forth earlier in this volume and will be repeated in "Best Techniques for Pain-Free Longevity," Chapter Thirty-One.

Now let us consider foods fit for the heart patient, and foods unfit for this class of patient.

Raw wheat germ contains the *natural* anti-clot ingredient that medical people prescribe *artificially* in the form of anti-coagulants. If you have a weak heart you should take on board every day of your life a small cereal-sized portion of raw wheat germ because of its alphatocopherol content which, in my opinion, is so far ahead of the medical anticoagulant drugs as not to be in the same league.

After every meal I advise all cardiac patients I know to take 200 International Units of vitamin E. Also, in my view, the use of 500 milligrams of vitamin C daily provides an anti-infection "cushion" needed in this polluted, ecologically substandard world.

I am of the opinion that on the eating level the best foods for the cardiac victim are, besides raw wheat germ (which must not be rancid—please note), a couple of tablespoonsful of lecithin granules daily, half a tablespoonful of yeast for its vitamin B factors, about the same amount of bone meal for the valuable absorbable and appropriable calcium it contains. The lecithin should be from soybeans preferably; and if one is an ethical vegetarian who will not touch animal products, a position I respect with all my heart, I advise whole barley as a substitute.

In addition to these products, I insist on at least one tablespoonful of soybean oil which has not been heat-processed but is cold pressed. In the absence of soybean oil I think safflower oil may be substituted.

An easy way to take everyday the foods that are right for the cardiac is I believe *the cereal way*. Merely throw together the foods mentioned above in a cereal bowl, as follows:

> Raw wheat germ, 2 to 6 tablespoonfuls
>
> Lecithin granules from soybeans, 2 tablespoonfuls
>
> Non-bitter yeast, one-half tablespoon
>
> Bone meal, one-half tablespoon

and add to all of it a full tablespoon of soybean oil, some sliced peaches, bananas, prunes or other fruit for taste and sweetening. Taking this with a little skimmed milk in the cereal bowl—and also some dried dates or figs if very hungry—will provide the nutritional needs of the cardiac patient provided he also takes 200 International Units of vitamin E after the meal. This means that 600 units of vitamin E, 200 after each meal, are consumed every day. Also, say at bedtime, one supplement of 500 mg. of vitamin C will provide the rest of what I think the heart-weak patient needs.

But there are some important "do-not-eat" items which I am firmly convinced the heart case must consider.

Eggs may be eaten only rarely. One egg once a week is all I ever approve for heart sufferers. I know about the "studies" which purport to show that eggs contain their own counteracting lecithin and therefore are good for heart victims. These people couldn't have had test cases in research groups the way I have had such controlled cases in tests and come to the same conclusion. I have found, at least by convincing empirical determinations, that eggs do indeed add to the blood cholesterol levels, that they do indeed impair the heart or the arteries leading thereto, and that although it is a fact that one's liver manufactures most of the cholesterol anyway, it is a still more pertinent fact that notwithstanding this the cardiac victim who consumes plenty of eggs suffers more than plenty of coronary occlusion attacks.

Consistent with the foregoing, people with heart problems should eat no hard margarine at all, no lard whatever, no butter except on the rarest occasions. They must forego all use of white granulated sugar. They must consider anything that emerges from the commercial bakeries as being off limits for them. Whole grain cereals are permitted. Whole grain breads from known sources may also be taken. But the cardiac can make better use of potatoes, fresh corn, brown rice or whole barley when he needs starchy foods.

Jams, jellies, anything sweetened with sugar should be avoided. Honey is better left to the bees. Sweetening, when craved, should come exclusively from fresh fruits or dried fruits if sun-dried, not chemically dried in sulfer baths or such. And drinks, when thirst beckons, should come altogether from slowly sucking on an orange, tomato, peach, persimmon or other watery fruit where the fluid is nonchlorinated or fluoridated or otherwise chemicalized.

(This need not be forever. If fluids are sharply held down in the abovementioned fashion for say a six-month period while the strengthening drills and nerve-unpinching routines given in this book are followed, heart repair will have gone on without the obstructions that careless, unknowing eaters usually place in the path of self-healing, and then the heart will be sufficiently strong to let you make your happy and well-loved violations from time to time.)

Besides the breakfast cereal dish recommended as daily fare, the cardiac patient should have raw salad vegetable plates as frequently as he desires. No condiments, however, are permitted. Salt especially is prohibited. Milk and general dairy products are not advised except for the bit of skimmed milk with the morning heart-feeding dish.

Heart cases also do well with a daily 15-minute exposure to the sun at permitted times, that is, before 10:00 in the morning and after 4:00 in the afternoon. In the evening, whenever possible, they should walk with bare feet on the earth or grass, or at least sit for a half hour with some part of their bare skin contacting the soil.

For the most part, meat proteins are ill-advised because of the contaminants which serve to obstruct healing. Procuring protein needs from sunflower seeds, peas, dry beans, coconut, almonds, avocados, wheat germ or whole wheat cereal, brown rice, etc. is a better way to serve and strengthen a weak heart.

***

The Diet to Normalize Kidneys and Bladder

Our effort in this very valuable diet is to get rid of soft, swollen, water-logged cells that are very vulnerable to disease, and exchange them in the organism for hardy dry cellular entities that are more nearly immune to disease.

The all-too-commonly heard advice to drink glass after glass of water, which in my firm opinion is a nonscientific piece of gibberish that is ruinous to human kidneys, should at once be ignored by those with kidney problems. And to an even greater degree, those with problems of the urinary bladder, those who rise at night too often or urinate too frequently during the day, and especially those unfortunates who cannot contain their urine and are embarrassed victims of "dribbling," should read and carefully heed what is written here about *nondrinking of nearly all fluids* for a time.

When I instructed patients with kidney and/or bladder difficulties to stop consuming all soups, sodas, water, tea and coffee I obtained the best results of all. For one full week they were required to give their kidney-bladder-urinary apparatus a rest. Any fluid they ingested was by way of small—very small—pieces of watery fruits such as peaches, nectarines, persimmons, oranges, tomatoes—all of which were slowly sucked, never guzzled rapidly. Then I fell upon an even more beneficial idea. For a week they were instructed to spoon every drop of fluid that went into their system. Never take a drink of anything, as such. Just take a spoonful out of a glass or cup, one spoon at a time. This worked wonders.

In Pavlov's *The Work of the Digestive Organs,* the great Russian physiologist made it clear that one does not need fluids to help in swallowing mealtime solid foods. "Foods with much water," he wrote, "cause only a scanty flow of saliva." And in the same work he makes clear my own thesis and emphasis on the value of the fluid*less* eating regimen. "Dry food excites a large flow of saliva," he said. Thus one need but chew each mouthful well and there will be enough saliva for the proper swallowing mechanism.

The great thing here is that when no outside water or soup or coffee is taken with the meal, the dry and solid nutrients are not thinned down or watered down. They are taken into the digestive system whole. They are fully nutritious instead of being attenuated and weakened by an admixture of inert water.

The best thing I ever learned to do *for kidneys,* next to finding nerve pressures on pathways to these organs and re-establishing a free flow of energizing and self-healing nerve impulses by correcting vertebral subluxations, was to give them a rest. Often it was the first rest of their lives. It was so extraordinarily easy to do. Merely stop the drinking of *anything.* Everything and anything. No fluid intake at all for a week. Dry solid food, yes. Water or soups or sodas or hot drinks, no. If you have poorly functioning kidneys just try this for only one week.

The ideal diet for kidney sufferers in my opinion is this: Depend entirely upon food intake for your body's fluid needs. Take, for example, such common items as carrots, turnips and apples. In a pound of any of these there are about 14 ounces of fluid. Not the city water kind of chemicalized inert fluid but the most purified fluid imaginable. Even in a pound of green peas you have about 12 ounces of good rich fluid. In tomatoes it is nearly all fluid, and in raw cabbage the fluid content is only slightly less. Bananas, dry as they seem, contain around 12 ounces of pure water to the pound.

All I require kidney sufferers to do is stop guzzling water or taking fluids into their system. With the foods mentioned above so rich in fluid content, plus frequent helpings of raw salad vegetables, one is never thirsty because of the great *natural* fluid intake. With this diet real thirst only rears its head if sharp spices are used—and they are forbidden. But even then, if thirsty, sucking the fluid out of an orange or tomato *slowly* will quench thirst in kidney cases better than quaffing two glassfuls of water at a single downpouring.

For bladder cases it is almost the same, but not quite. Since drinks overstretch the blood vessels and overirritate the weak valvular outlet of the urinary bladder, I have found the following diet plan best for virtually all cases.

Pour some boiling water over a cereal dish containing sliced fruits such as pears, apples, peaches and plums. Cover the dish for a few hours and begin drinking it a spoonful at a time after it has cooled. When cutting up the fruit, use every part of each item: seeds in the cores, all the skins, everything gets soaked in the hot water.

For three days all fluids are eliminated if they are not from vital, organic, natural foods. The water in which the fresh fruits have been soaked is drunk by the spoonful, only a few spoonfuls at a time every two hours or so. And even then only if there is thirst.

This gives the urinary bladder a rest from ordinary day-to-day functioning. After six in the evening no drinks of any kind are allowed, not even by the spoonful. If very greatly thirsty, merely gargle a mouthful of water but do not swallow it. After three days of this the diet requires you to quench thirst only from melons, persimmons, tomatoes, apples, pears and peaches or nectarines. All, you will note, will be fluid from vital *natural* sources. No soups or coffee or any other beverage is permitted for at least a two-week period.

After this two- or three-week period, more or less regular eating may be resumed, but with this restriction. No glassful or cupful of water or beverage is ever drunk. If taken at all, it is sipped, and always sipped very slowly. No watery soups are ever permitted. Cereals, if desired, must be whole grain cereals and taken with as little skimmed milk as possible. It is really better to mix a cereal with as much yogurt or clabber or sour milk as will make the item edible or swallowable. I encourage the use of yogurt or clabber for its value in laying into the digestive apparatus an intestinal flora of lactic acid bacilli which will protect against fungi or deep-seated fungus infection.

One final note of extreme value to kidney problem cases, and another for bladder problem victims.

Kidneys

A single glassful of raw beet juice, freshly squeezed and taken only a spoonful at a time all through one full day. One teaspoonful of this raw beet juice about every ten minutes from morning until night. Nothing else that one day. The urine may turn very red, which is natural and not at all alarming. The beet juice is not flavored or spiced in any way. Do not drink beet juice in great quantities; it is too powerful and can do harm. This plan of spooning beet juice into the system for one day somehow, in a way not yet clearly understood, clears debris out of human kidneys and is a kind of restorative new lease on life. Kidney life. This may be repeated every two months; that is, one full day of only spoon-fed beet juice every 60 days.

Bladder

A spoonful of watercress-soaked water every few minutes during the day acts as a powerful *natural* diuretic. Alternating this with a day on watermelon has given relief and benefits to bladder cases in my experience when nothing else was able to help. Merely soak a fresh supply of watercress in boiling water for an hour, or until cool enough to drink, and take a spoonful of this every hour or so. Do this for one full day from early morning until sunset, not later. On the following day take a small cube of watermelon into your mouth every few minutes all day long, just for one day. The amount of fluid you will void during this period will amaze you. It is a first-rate cleansing plan. Coupled with the important nerve-unpinching program set forth in this book, it will mean that you are doing for your kidneys and bladder more than any other healing plan known to me can ever or has ever done.

***

The Diet to Naturally Help Emphysema and Asthma

I believe that the best way to start supplying useful and workable information on the level of *foods for emphysema and asthma* is to set down a *No List* and a *Yes List*.

List of Foods to Avoid
 1. Meat fats
 2. Butter
 3. Lard
 4. Hard margarine
 5. Sweet cream
 6. Sour cream
 7. Hard cheeses
 8. Oils and oily foods
 9. Salt and salty foods
10. Herring and fatty fish
11. Sugar
12. Fatty vegetables such as avocados, olives and coconuts
13. Eggs
14. Nearly all cooked foods

   All of the items mentioned tend to form an injurious over-supply of mucus in the human system. Mucus in excess is the hallmark of asthma and emphysema. This applies also to bronchitis and related chest or lung problems. If you stop fueling the system with foods that tend to form too much mucus, you are being good to yourself by stopping the intake of injurious substances *at source*.

List of Foods to Consume
 1. Berries
 2. Fresh pineapple
 3. Tomatoes
 4. Lemons
 5. Oranges
 6. Grapefruits
 7. Limes
 8. Strawberries, especially
 9. Most sour fruits
10. Acerola berries as leading source of vitamin C (ascorbic acid)

All of these items tend to dissolve accumulations of mucus in the system. Working contrarily to mucus forming foods, these mucus solvent foods have the happy faculty of dissolving the mucus overloads that bother emphysematous and asthmatic people. By doing both things—eliminating the mucus formers and consuming the mucus solvents, the one suffering from the plagues of coughing and wheezing due to asthma and emphysema usually sees a great degree of precious results in no more than a week.

The citrus fruits should be eaten whole, not fragmented in the form of juice. An orange, for example, should be consumed entirely—pulp, juice, bioflavonoids, the whole thing. So also should grapefruits, limes, tomatoes and the like be eaten in their entirety. Note that animals in the untamed (instinctual) state eat the whole carcass of the hunted-down animal; not merely the muscle meat in the form of steaks that humans prefer, but the organs and glands and entrails and all.

Having read the foregoing about foods that tend to form mucus and those that tend to dissolve mucus, put it aside for the nonce and apply yourself to the following.

The best diet to *naturally help emphysema and asthma* is in my tried-and-tested opinion, *the exclusive fruit diet.*

I have called this The Primate Diet. Here is the reason: I have no personal doubt that man as a living biped began life in the tropics. In the tropics, fruit was abundant and fruit is what he ate originally. Only fruit. Then he came to realize the enormous value and versatility of the apposable thumb, and he began to wander. Wandering out of the tropics he found fruits not so abundant and began to eat vegetables indigenous to the areas of his new abode. His body adapted to vegetables, and later even to flesh foods when he wandered still farther north and had to depend on hunting and fishing.

But his original diet was the fruit diet. It is still the *primal diet,* the one man's body is naturally most accustomed to. In times of doubt, when doctors and all about you are baffled by your illness, go on the fruit diet for a week and note the near-magic changes that occur.

Every case of emphysema and asthma that I have ever instructed to go on a week, sometimes two, of nothing but fruits, has profited to some degree, often with great unexpected benefits.

After a week of The Primate Diet, eating as much as you desire of only fruits at any one sitting—but trying to make the meals small even if you require six instead of three meals daily—set before you the list of mucus-forming foods and avoid them.

If dessert is required at mealtimes, only the foods from the list of mucus-solvent foods should be taken. I have seen especially gratifying results from the consumption of fresh strawberries, possibly because they are alone among food that are known to contain organic salicylates—the active ingredient in aspirins, anacins, etc. They should never be seasoned or sweetened, only eaten whole after washing. Honey should not be employed. *Sugar never at any time for any reason whatsoever.*

Making an entire meal of only a dish of fresh strawberries is recommended.

All asthma and emphysema cases must—positively must—have nerves that may be pinched unblocked and unpinched. The drills in Chapter Thirty-One will show you how to achieve this. If there is halted or improper conductivity of the nervous system's nerve impulses to the chest area, then even if you follow all diet instructions to the letter the body will lack the healing power to mend its damages. Thus you must, as the chiropractic doctors have it, *turn on the power.* If you cannot quite unblock all of your own nerve pressures with the drills presented in this book, have a chiropractic doctor do it for you a time or two and then proceed on your own.

One further item for asthma and emphysema cases: No cold foods or drinks. No drinks at all, but only short and slow sips of fluids when thirsty. Attend to these instructions for a fortnight and learn again the joy of breathing health.

***

The Diet for Gallstones

This one I call the whilom diet. I mean this in the sense that it is a *sometime* diet. When it works the results are little short of incredible. When it doesn't it is a sheer waste of time, but with no harm done the body in the least.

These stones, or calculi, are composed of different material. My experience has been that if the accumulation or concretion is made up of material that can be pulverized, or that can be made to fall apart like grains of sand, it is a gallstone which may yield to the following diet. If, however, what is termed a biliary cholelithiasis is a hard, stone-like form of gallstone, it cannot be dissolved or made to come apart and leave the system in little granules.

In any case, I believe the diet that follows is worth a try. And although I do not present it with the assurance that goes with the presentation of other diets in this section—and this is simply and honestly because I have not known it to work uniformly and beneficially as I've seen the others work—I feel it earns a place here.

You rise in the morning and eat only fruit. Mixed with the variety of grapes, peaches, pears and apples you try to take also a small avocado or half of a large one. Just before noontime you eat about eight ounces of plain yogurt, then no food at all after mid-day.

At about six o'clock immerse yourself into a hot bath. I seldom recommend a very hot bath, but do for this program. The idea is to make it as hot as can be comfortably borne. Heat tends to dilate all parts of the body as it expands even the steel rails of the railroad track. Immersed up to your neck in the hot water, the common bile duct that leads from the gall bladder hopefully will dilate and get large enough to let the gallstones pass out.

At 7 p.m. you go to bed and must be prepared to lie *only on your right side* until the next morning. At your bedside you have prepared and waiting to be consumed a *full pint of olive oil* and a *full cup of freshly squeezed lemon juice.*

Every 15 minutes take four tablespoonfuls of olive oil and one tablespoonful of lemon juice.

In about three hours you will have consumed all the oil and lemon juice—all this while lying on the right side.

Following this you go to sleep on the right side. In the morning upon rising you feel an urge to defecate and, if this program succeeds in your case, the stones will be evacuated through the bowels.

Then, as one patient wrote to me, you will have cause to celebrate your "coming out party."

In this program the oil activates the elimination of gallstones in two ways: First, it tends to expand the duct through which the stones must pass. Second, it lubricates the lining of the duct and makes it *sufficiently slippery* to let the stones slide out painlessly. The lemon juice acts to hold down nausea, for that much oil tends to nauseate. Even with that cupful of lemon juice there may be a bit of nausea and even a little cramping, but not often and not much.

Following this program, and the passage of the gallstones, it should be borne in mind that the expanded duct ought to be allowed to contract back to normal dimensions. Therefore, it is urgent that *all* fats and oils and greases be avoided for about a month or six weeks.

This is not by my own research in any way. All that I have personally found beneficial to add was the fruit breakfast with a bit of oily food (avocado or coconut) as preparation for the program, and especially the physiologically correct immersion in a hot bath to prepare the duct by expanding it.

What follows, however, sometimes works as well in evacuating gallstones and is decidedly easier to do. Merely boil beet leaves and eat them. Not the beets themselves or the stalks, but only the leaves. We do not know why this works. But by trial and error we do know empirically that it does work with great frequency.

Devote one day to eating beet leaves. Nothing there to hurt you if it doesn't quite accomplish what you want. Boil a large quantity of these leaves, do not season them, eat a satisfying portion of this three times during the one day of the test. People who have had what is called "a gall bladder attack" and were told to consume these boiled beet leaves can attest to the efficacy of the program. Often it is hardly short of miraculous.

In either the olive oil-lemon juice program or the beet leaves approach to gallstones and gall bladder problems, a repeat performance for one day is advised in six months if all the stones are not evacuated or if all the gall duct congestion/inflammation has not been assuaged.

*****

The Diet to Balance the Blood Chemistry (Mono-Diet)

In all the years of attending to the sick and researching natural avenues of self-healing, five definite aids for ailing persons have impressed themselves on my consciousness.

It is astonishing, really. No matter how much is done to help a sick person back to health, I have found that I cannot *reasonably* expect him or her to get truly well unless all five of these discovered aids have been attended to. If two are met but three of these irreducible needs are not, the sick person may improve but will not return to full health.

What then are these five absolute requirements for human health? Note them well.

Chemical balance. The blood chemistry of a person must be in harmonious balance or sickness will rear its head.

Mechanical balance. Besides being a chemical factory the body is also a machine, a mechanical contraption. Like any machine it must be in proper mechanical adjustment. No one but a fool would expect a machine that is not in mechanical adjustment to work right. In his great book, *Body Mechanics in Health and Disease,* the eminent Dr. Joel Goldthwait, former president of the American Orthopedic Association, says that the first thing to do in sickness, before diets or surgery or drugs are sought, is to put the body back into mechanical shape "so that all the organs may have the chance to do jobs for which they were intended." And he goes on to say that to first take drugs or the other medical things is to "court disaster" because, without the body's being in correct mechanical adjustment, it is "not possible for the various organs to do the work they were intended to do."

The other three absolute requirements for real health, as I have researched them and proved them, are these: *Gravity factors*—paying every day the toll that living against gravity exacts from us every day. *Oxygenation*—improving the breathing apparatus so that we might better "make do" with the poor oxygen quality of our polluted atmosphere. *Nervous tension*—how to siphon off the accumulated tensions of our rush-rush, hurry-flurry world.

All of the forgoing three are adequately covered in this volume. The unutterably important requirement of *Mechanical Balance* is fully explained, with plenty of drills and self-help techniques, in Chapter Twelve under the heading of "Best Exercises for Pain-Free Longevity."

For attaining *Chemical Balance* I have never met anything to equal the value of the "Mono-Diet."

Following the Mono-Diet is almost an assurance that any chemical imbalance in the bloodstream and body chemistry will after a reasonable period become a relatively pure blood stream and a balanced body chemistry. There are good reasons why this is so.

It is fair to say that most ills flowing from inner chemical imbalance come from bad combinations of foods, eating dishes not compatible with each other. Combinations that cause gas, belching, acid regurgitations and other symptoms that indicate wrongly put-together foods.

Mono-Diet is the answer to all this. The genius and virtue of Mono-Diet is that it avoids combinations altogether.

The best combination is no combination at all.

Therein lies the head and front of the Mono-Diet program. It is the program of eating only one food at a time. As much as one may desire of that food, but only the one food at the one sitting.

You desire citrus fruits? Eat all the oranges you want for breakfast—but only oranges. No combinations to worry about. Oranges combine excellently with themselves. You like bananas? Consume all the well-chewed and insalivated bananas for lunch—but only bananas. There you have taken care of a fruit breakfast and a starch lunch. You like sunflower seeds, whole or ground? Take as much as you like of this protein for your evening meal. Chew well enough to mix with sufficient saliva and all will go well digestively.

There is physiological astuteness behind this. Most people eat far too much. One reason for this is that they eat a variety of foods at a meal, and when full to bursting with the main course and certainly should not take anything more on board, they can be tempted on a higher taste plane with ice cream or stewed fruits. With the magic of Mono-Diet, however, all this seems to be obviated. You can eat only so much of oranges or of bananas at any one time, no matter how greatly you like oranges or bananas. Your own digestive safety valve is at work protecting you from indiscretions. When you have consumed three oranges, you stop. When you have taken three or four bananas for lunch, you quit. The digestive organs do not overwork. They are never overloaded. They have no problem of dealing with incompatible combinations. Possibly for the first time in their history as an adult digestive machine, they rest properly even while performing their work properly.

Here then follows the wonderful Mono-Diet. It will permit you to eat as many as 21 different foods in a week if you choose. Merely select a different food each time three times a day for the full week. If at the same time you attend to the drills in Chapter Thirty-One that teach you how to unpinch any nerves to the digestive organs that may be pinched and thus unable to transmit functional power to such organs, in a reasonably short time your digestion should be a matter of wellbeing and happiness.

NOTE: As a gift and payment for your observance of this extraordinarily helpful Mono-Diet, I will set forth here, by way of pre-payment, a delicious dessert that you may have and that, surprisingly enough, fits exactly into the plan because it is a one-food item fancied up to resemble more. It's "ice cream." Do you like ice cream? Here is how to do it and still be on the Mono-Diet magic. Remove the skins from a half dozen or more well-ripened bananas and place the fruit in the freezing receptacle of your refrigerator. When frozen hard, cut them fine, place them in your blender and whirl them up at a high speed. That is all. They whip up into a banana ice cream both delicious and nutritious. And sugarless. Not a single item has been added. Pure bananas. Bananas with their own natural sweetness. The perfect "ice cream."

Food Items Properly Fitting into Mono-Diet Plan

Proteins	Starches	Fruits	Neutral Foods
Wheat germ	Bananas	Pears	Broccoli
Sunflower seeds	Potatoes	Apples	Asparagus
Whole barley	Corn	Persimmons	Cabbage
Brown rice	Chestnuts	Grapes	Lettuce
Peas	Squash	Tomatoes	Chard
Dry beans	Oats	Peaches	Cucumbers
Legumes	Pumpkin	Plums	Okra
Avocados	Wheatena	Pineapples	Boiled onions
Walnuts		Grapefruit	Zucchini
Almonds		Oranges	Eggplant
Coconut		Nectarines	Kale
Soybeans			
Buttermilk			
Cottage cheese			

Try this Mono-Diet for just a single week and note the results. Try not to cheat, for it will be a self-infliction and not at all self-serving. After a week, if as enthusiastic as most people are, try another week of it. An entire month of this no-combination eating plan will reestablish normality in just about any digestive ailment that can be reversed—provided, as always, there is no nerve pressure to the digestive organs and the stomach, liver, pancreas, intestines are receiving their required flow of nerve impulses through unblocked nerves to energize and direct them in their operations. (If in doubt about this, follow the instructions in Chapter Thirty-One.)

If you are one of those without patience to follow any program for as long as a week or two, here is a compromise plan to help you make it. At the evening meal, after having eaten only a single food for breakfast and lunch, add as large a plate as you can consume of the foods listed *neutral*.

This will give you something to look forward to all day. I advise that you make the evening meal your protein meal. Say you are having two ounces of sunflower seeds or almonds, an excellent choice. Along with this you may then take a large plate full of cucumbers, lettuce, some boiled onions, some steamed zucchini squash, even a few spears of canned asparagus. Add no seasoning aside from lemon juice.

Then, as a further treat, you have that gloriously delicious banana "ice cream" I've included as your bonus. And you will still be right on the Mono-Diet plan. How much do you want to be coddled, anyway! I advise that you save the banana "ice cream" for a bedtime snack. Do these things for a month, or even less, and have tests made of your blood chemistry if you are in doubt. You will find that you have been very, very good to yourself.

***

The Diet for Migraines and Other Headaches

In Chapter Thirty-One of this book I have given some excellent nerve-pinching techniques which are often very beneficial for migraine headaches. They call for enclosing the side of the neck in your cupped open hands and lifting the head off the shoulders. The lift is straight upward and a bit forward. This tends to traction the neck and take nerve pressure away. It is a manner of unpinching nerve pressures in the neck that has been found admirably helpful in nearly all kinds of headaches.

Once this is attended to—or while doing the nerve-unpinching drills for the neck—the entire system must be cleansed and purified if migraines are to go away and stay away.

There are various approaches to this. I have tried many, discarded most, retained some. The very best of all plans for migraines on *the diet level* follow.

A three-day fast is almost a necessity. Often it has to be continued for as many as ten days. Nothing at all is eaten. Drinks are limited to a bit of water whenever there is thirst. No fluid is taken into the system unless it fills a physiological need—unless it is triggered by actual thirst, that is.

The best plan is to go to bed and stay there for the time of the fast. Stay there and do nothing at all. The reason for this is that we can in this way conserve the energy otherwise expended in activities. The energy thus conserved is used by the self-healing body to repair the cellular damages of the organism, clear the bloodstream of toxic debris, step up the metabolic process. If serious about this, I can give no better advice than to carve a three-day period or even ten-day period out of your life exclusively for the purpose of rebuilding the body. Stay in bed and do nothing; no reading, writing, television viewing or other things which utilize energy. Most of all, no talking. Just pull down the shades, thus darkening the room to save the energy used in accommodating to light, and do nothing.

Watch the tongue. If it coats rapidly, keep up the fast until it clears and becomes cherry red or pink. Don't mind the foul odor that exudes from you; that's the poison being driven out by exhalations. Sip water whenever thirsty, sleep as much as you can, suspend exercises for the time of the fast, take a 15-minute sunbath if you can each day earlier than ten in the morning and later than four in the afternoon.

Following the fast, take only diluted orange juice or tomato juice, about an ounce or two every two hours the first day. Equal portions of fruit juice and water are advised. Sip every drop slowly. On the second day following the fast take undiluted sips of fruit juice plus small portions of steamed zucchini squash—no seasoning added.

After these two preparatory days go on the strict Primate Diet for as long as you wish, hopefully until all signs of headache are gone. This diet, as you may recall, is the diet our ancient ancestors first thrived on—nothing but fruit. Choose the fruits most tasteful to your palate. Eat your fill of them. The watery fruits should preferably be taken slowly, not permitting the fluid content to enter the system all at once. Sucking the juice out of an orange or tomato is better than eating the fruit whole. When the fluid is extracted, however, the whole fruit should be consumed.

***

The Diet for Soothing and Nourishing the Nervous System

Since the nervous system is actually in control of all other systems of the human body, everything we eat nourishes or does ill first of all to our nerve structures.

But, as in nearly all things, some of the things we may do every day are very good and helpful and nourishing for the nervous system, others very bad. If sunflower seeds or almonds are eaten instead of meat to fill our protein needs, for example, it may appear that the digestive system profits most but in reality it is the nervous system that derives greatest benefit. Why is this so? It is a rather complicated explanation. Reduced to simplicity, meat proteins bear contaminants within them, nuts do not. The diseases that the slaughtered animal has had are in the meat fiber. The six ounces or so of watery element in an eight-ounce serving of steak or chops is polluted water when seen in this realistic and purely scientific context. The pollutants irritate the nerve endings *at the very least*. Thus, since nerves direct and energize and control all else in the body, everything else suffers. Yet none of this harmful side effect ensues from the consumption of nuts or peas or avocados to fill our protein needs.

When is a food—any food—truly good for you? Are there any criteria by which we can judge a food's goodness or badness for the human body? Thomas Henry Huxley laid it out for us rather neatly. Let us examine Huxley's tests for determining whether a food is fit for human use:

> *Appearance:* Does the item of food look like it can be eaten?

Odor: Does it smell as though it is fit for eating?

Taste: Is it pleasant or offensive to our taste buds?

Alas, our food processing and packaging fancy fellows have robbed us of the validity of these simple tests. They can artificially color a food that looks unfit for use and make it seem glowing with attractiveness. They can doctor up a foul-smelling food to give it a heavenly odor. They can *and do* make ill-tasting foods assume the flavor of ambrosia by adding chemicals and carcinogenic flavorings.

I would update Huxley's criteria as follows. Can a food be eaten raw? Does it need to be prepared (thus altered)? Is cooking essential? Could an undomesticated animal, or any animal for that matter, lacking human facilities of the kitchen, make use of it? If a food is not edible as it comes from nature, and man has to have something to do with it to make it usable, it at once becomes suspect. Anything that man packages or processes for profit, man too often destroys, denudes, denatures, devitalizes or just plain poisons. Think of foods that can be eaten as nature gives them to us: apples, pears, melons, all fruits, all nuts, all vegetables, wheat and other cereals, even meat and fish and eggs. But not boxed and artificially sugared-flavored-toasted-puffed cereals. Not tinned or canned goods of any kind. Not soups or coffee or soda drinks.

Among foods that *most* soothe and nourish the nerves I would name wheat germ and whole grains. All foods that deliver cellulose or roughage to the system ensure a good peristaltic action and thus proper elimination of poisons out of the system after the needed nutrients are absorbed. If not enough wheat germ is available I certainly would recommend (in this imperfect world) tablets of vitamin B from wheat germ sources.

Because foods containing the B-vitamins are good nourishers of the nervous system I encourage the consumption of green leafy vegetables (kale, mustard greens, broccoli, chard, etc.) and also the yellow vegetables. Among my favorite desserts, if indeed any dessert is needed, is a baked apple, unsugared, nonhoneyed, only with raisins added. This has good vitamin B content, as also does the avocado, apricot, pineapple. Tomatoes, cantaloupes, prunes are also among my favorite B-vitamin foods, thus nourishing for the nerve pathways of the body.

For best nerve integrity I would advise small meals, never heavy and large ones. Eat six times a day if necessary, but make the meals small ones.

Facing our imperfect world as we do, and having to "make do" with it, in the absence of good B-vitamin foods I would certainly take a full tablespoon of powdered (debittered) yeast every day.

By all means, for the sake of a good functioning and non-irritated nervous system, I would advise keeping the protein consumption low, very low. A couple of ounces a day are more than sufficient. I have been writing this for years. Now, just lately, people in "the scientific community" are beginning to ask where the strong ox and horse get their strength on a low protein intake. Notwithstanding this, you will probably still pick up articles (claiming *scientificness)* which will counsel you to take plenty of protein *to keep up your strength.*

In addition to the foregoing ways to soothe and nourish the nervous system, that is, the use of *wheat germ, whole grains, vitamin B, green and yellow vegetables, fruits rich in B-vitamins such as apricots, pineapples, tomatoes, prunes, baked apples, a daily tablespoonful of yeast, small meals* and LOW PROTEIN INTAKE AND NO SOUPS OR FLUIDS OR CANNED GOODS, I would add the following safeguards.

Avoid eating fruit skins. I do not believe the body contains enzymes to properly and fully break down skins, thus we see wholly undigested tomato skins in the stool from time to time. The skins cover impermeably what is the good nourishing food underneath, but were not themselves intended to be eaten.

In general, if you need to cook it, overlook it.

This is subject to exceptions of course, because of our imperfect world. But, for the most part, if you eat foods raw your system will thrive better on them. The word "raw" is not in fact a correct one to use. Nothing is raw, actually. It has all been "cooked" in the laboratory of nature as it grew and was warmed by the sun's rays, nourished by the earth and rains, filtered and refined and prepared through the roots and branches.

As additional protection I favor everyone's taking a multi-vitamin tablet (which is at the same time also multi-mineral) every day. If our soils were better (less overworked and impoverished) I would not advise this. But even with the best diet of well-chosen fruits, vegetables, nuts, grains, the realities of my experience with sick people force me to add multi-vitamins-minerals for extra protection.

A good rule to remember is that overeating is overliving. The explanation can be a little tricky. Suffice it to say that when you overeat you also overmetabolize; and when you overmetabolize you *overlive*—meaning you use up your capacities sooner and thus *use yourself up* in shorter time.

If you go on a fast, never make it a mere one-day fast. Some people pride themselves on fasting one day a week. They are really uninformed people, in my opinion. The body is geared to eating, not to noneating. Whenever one fasts therefore, one sustains a slight neurological shock by *ungearing* the system. So if a person recognizes the value of fasting, which is great indeed, he should go on a fast that is long enough to accomplish some good. The one-day-a-week fast merely teases the system back and forth and cannot be advised as doing any real good.

As indicated elsewhere, no cold plunges are to be indulged in as a daily "health habit" because that also is a shock to the nervous system. Although the cold plunge has nothing to do with diet, and this section is about diets that soothe and nourish the nervous system, I mention it because it "unsoothes" and also "unnourishes" many a nervous system.

Permit me to return, and to underline, what I wrote previously about the value of proteins in wheat germ or nuts or peas over the proteins resident in flesh products. The flesh itself, as indicated, is contaminated with diseases present or past. The three-quarters watery part of the meat or fish is polluted water because of its very relationship with the flesh. As one writer put it, the water in a steak is dirty water, while the water in protein-rich peas or dry beans or wheat is clean water. Flesh protein burdens the kidneys which must filter out of the system such toxic waste products. In nonflesh proteins, however, it is all clean and not in any wise a burden on the heart, the kidneys, most of all the nerve cells.

But—and I must in truth interpose an important "but" here. Lest one get unduly worried and deeply disturbed about an occasional indiscretion in flesh-eating, *I believe there is actual value in violating the rules from time to time.* This is a heresy that many of my colleagues will not countenance in me. All the same, I know from many testings and "adventures in research" that the human body was made to handle toxins. It was not altogether made to be toxin-free.

I do not advise anyone to make his bloodstream and body chemistry entirely pure and toxin-free. My reason rests on all-too-frequent and disturbing observations. Over the decades I'd seen people who never violated eating rules and had what could be called a pure bloodstream, free of toxic elements. These people were too vulnerable to disease in this unsafe world. If they chanced to enter a restaurant and be served anything at all that was not exactly pure, their systems, having been untrained to handle toxins, revolted and became gravely ill. The same food, served to people whose systems were accustomed to handling toxins daily, did not cause illness at all. In extreme cases, the pure of body even died while the impure lived.

Consequently, my advice must be this: *Don't make yourself too pure.* Do not permit your system to forget how to handle toxins. The rule is as follows, I have found. Your good health is not the result of what you do once in a while but of what you do most of the time. If you violate once in a while, that's really insurance in this polluted order of things that you won't get sick if inadvertently consuming a toxic-laden food.

I relate very happily to vegetarians, respecting them highly. But I have not failed to notice (as a doctor and observant researcher) that if they "break over" in the least they are sick the next day with running noses, coughs, fevers, all kinds of symptoms. Some violate in so small a degree as eating a slice of bakery-made bread and suffer the following day. Others who violate all the time eat bread (and worse) and feel fine.

To repeat: Your health will come from what you do most of the time, not from what you do once in a while. If you behave most of the time and kick over the traces or rules now and then, you will enjoy good health, I have discovered. I myself, the author of this book, almost purposely violate the well-understood rules of health just because I do not want my body to forget how to metabolize protein overuse and toxic waste products. Going on lecture tours as I frequently do, if the ladies of the reception committee for the visiting speaker have worked half the day preparing pressed duck or pheasant under glass, I am not about to become so uncivilized as to tell them "I eat only lettuce and tomatoes."

Why do I write all this?

I write to unfold the little-understood potentials of the body's genius for self-healing. Just give the body half a chance and it will make itself well unless the breakdown is so deep that the trouble is irreversible. Fortunately, most conditions are quite reversible if you remove the obstructions to self-healing.

Chief among obstructions to self-healing are nerve pressures, so what soothes the nerve cells most is to unpinch the nerve pathways of irritating occlusions. Read Chapter Thirty-One; then do the unpinching drills.

Reread this section many times and learn "by heart" what to eat, and what to avoid, so that your nervous system, true master system of the body, gets soothed and properly nourished.

***

The Compromise Diet
for Those Who Feel They Can't Follow Diets

In dealing with many hundreds of sick people the doctor who faces reality finds that there are some who just cannot undertake diets.

A small number cannot follow any kind of diet at all.

They have reasons why they cannot. Sometimes the reasons are mere self-acquitting rationalizations. Sometimes they are obviously and painfully self-indulgent. Often they are sound reasons, at least to the patient. In many instances the reasons are adequate because to him or her the business needs or social requirement to do and be like everyone else outweighs the requirement to lose weight or be well.

Here are some of the reasons given me over the years, so that you may recognize them in yourself or in friends who are sure they cannot diet.

"Whenever I quit coffee or cut down sharply on food, I get headachy and am not fit to live with."

"Nature must have meant me to be too fat (or skinny) because when I attempt to change it I get sick, whereas this way I enjoy good health."

"Let's face it—I just plain like eating and won't give up the joy of at least one or two good meals a day; the tasty things feel so good going down!"

"If I didn't take that martini with my business associates at lunch, or if I ate differently from them, I'd become a pariah instead of one of them, and it would cost me sales."

There is a saying that what can't be cured must be endured. Facing reality, then, those who cannot be made to diet must be permitted not to diet. But what about a kind of circuitous route for them? How about reaching their needs roundaboutly and helping them also?

Thinking about this, I came up with a plan. It was a scheme whereby I might be able to help even the nondieters gather up a good dose of that health that's waiting to be claimed by nearly everyone.

It would not be the very best way; but in extremity even second-choice health is better than no health. In the land where all are blind, goes the saying, even the one-eyed man is great.

So—for those of you who must violate the rules and disciplines of dieting—or think you must—hearken to what follows.

I have devised an eating plan that does not interfere with your mealtime schedules after breakfast. It is only the breakfast that I want you to give attention to. At this morning meal I mean to lay into your body very nearly all the fortifying and health-building substances the organism needs. It will be such a beautifully and bountifully balanced meal that even if you violate the rest of the day, as I expect you will, the one meal will keep you going in relative health.

Sounds good, doesn't it?

All right? Ready?

On rising take one multi-vitamin-mineral tablet or capsule plus one vitamin C capsule of 500 mg. Instead of water or fruit juice, swallow the vitamins with several spoonfuls of plain yogurt. That's the first thing you do.

Then you go about your business of shaving, bathing, exercising (I hope!), dressing and all the rest. In this way some little time has elapsed since you took the vitamins and minerals, the latter containing iron which must have a bit of time to be absorbed.

Your breakfast dish will be a whopper. A big dish indeed. Into a cereal bowl you pour as much raw wheat germ as you generally consume in any cereal equivalent. In place of say oatmeal or corn flakes or Wheatena, make it four or six ounces of wheat germ. To this you add several ingredients that will sustain you and *healthify* you. You may like them. But even if you don't, this is the one time you will be asked to be *not so self-indulgent* and discipline yourself a mite.

Have ready at your elbow (from the health food store or supermarket) a supply of the following:

Yogurt—not fancied up with fruit, just plain.

Soybean Lecithin—bottled in granule form.

Bone Meal—available in any health food store.

Powdered Yeast—ditto.

Fresh Fruit—slice any kind you desire.

Orange Juice or Apple Juice—as desired.

Soybean Oil—must be cold pressed, not heated.

Now, to the bowl of raw wheat germ you add about two tablespoonfuls of the soybean lecithin granules, one tablespoon of powdered yeast (the debittered kind), a half tablespoon of bone meal, even a little honey if you like. Mix all of this well with enough yogurt to give it the consistency of mush or tapioca—some even refer to it as custard. Add the sliced peaches, persimmons, pears, apples or whatever fruit you desire. If not sweet enough you may add more honey. If you insist on having your morning cereal in more liquid form than this, you may even pour skimmed milk into the bowl, enough to meet your taste.

Now, very slowly I hope, and masticating every mouthful thoroughly, *eat ye all of it*.

That's it—except for one more smallish thing.

You have consumed a bowl of wonderfully rich, powerful health-giving ingredients that even tastes good with all that sliced fruit and honey and nutty wheat germ. Now, just before you leave for your daily jousts with business colleagues, sip a small glass of apple juice or orange juice into which you have stirred a tablespoonful of soybean oil—cold-pressed soybean oil. In the absence of soybean oil, safflower will do. Mix the oil well by rapid stirring into the juice and sip all of it. Do not overlook this final drink, the "smallish thing" that caps the climax to the breakfast meal.

The soybean oil in conjunction with the raw wheat germ and lecithin granules at about the same time will afford you a protective base for the indiscretions of the day.

The yeast will give you the nerve nourishment needed for the business or social jousts.

The yogurt will tend to protect against intestinal infection.

The bone meal will mineralize the bones and provide both calcium and magnesium in best form possible.

All of it will generally see you through the day with more energy than is customarily provided by those de-energizing (truly enervating) business luncheons of martinis, meat and potatoes, apple pie and coffee.

Take this one big bowl of mixed ingredients for breakfast and *learn to like it* even if you don't at first. And do not fail to take that final drink of juice plus soybean oil. Even if you do not like oil, this is little enough to ask when it offers so much for you.

To anticipate your questions—no coffee, for breakfast, no. And no sugar in any form. But as large a bowl of this health mix as you like. And as much fruit as you want.

As a doctor I would wish that you eat properly all the rest of the day. But even if you don't, by adhering to this one breakfast program which is of course a kind of compromise diet, you will enjoy reasonably good health even if you violate. Certainly you will enjoy better health than if you took your regular bacon and egg, coffee, toast and jam breakfast in the usual way.

Chapter Thirty-One

The Best Exercises
for Pain-Free Longevity

Everyone wants to live a long time provided he can manage to have the years stretch before him without pains and discomforts.

The entire purpose of this chapter is precisely that of setting forth the ways to best achieve this goal. I have tried and discarded many forms of drills and exercises. I have kept and refined others. The best and most improved drills and exercises of greatest promise are here set forth.

First—of greatest importance—is the matter of removing nerve pressures from the spinal column and body generally. If you suffer pressures on nerve pathways you will be in pain and trouble no matter what else you do or don't do. So, keeping in mind that every spinal vertebra can be jolted or strained out of position and thereafter pinch vital nerves, thus preventing such pinched nerves from conducting functional Life Power to the organs which they serve, we concentrate on the best nerve-unpinching exercises.

Unpinching Nerve Pressures in the Neck

Sitting or standing, cup the sides of your neck in both open hands, the fingers just below the protruding mastoid bones and the palms below the jaws. Do not press toward the middle of the neck, for this may choke the jugular veins, but lift the head off the shoulders. Lift straight upward and a bit forward. As you lift in this way, turn the head as far as you can to the left, not slackening the lift as you turn. Then turn toward the right and continue lifting as you turn. Make the turn in each direction to the limit of motion. When you reach the limit of how far you can turn, keep lifting the head off the shoulder and try to get a little extra mobility by turning just a little farther. Do this especially at night, just before retiring. Do it several times during the day. When already in bed, lie flat on your back and take the strains of the day off your neck structures by lifting the head off the shoulders in the same way—this time lifting the head toward the headboard of the bed. (See Figure 1.) I have never known anything to equal this simple drill for nerve-unpinching exactitude. It will give you neck ease and pillow ease you never expected to have.

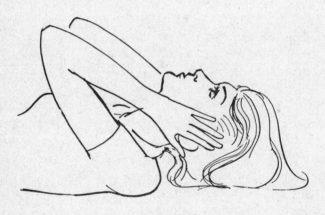

Figure 1

Unpinching Nerve Pressures in the Mid-Spine

Lie on the carpeted floor and raise your knees to the chest as you are flat on the back. (See Figure 2.) Bring the knees to the tips of the shoulders, or as near to the tips as you can. With a hand cupped over each knee press hard toward the shoulders, feeling the spine stretch and lengthen as you do this. Repeat as many times as you like, stopping when you feel vaguely tired.

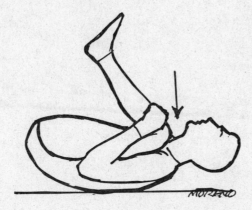

Figure 2

Another way that stretches the mid-spine and strongly tends to bring the vertebrae into alignment, thus unpinching nerves, is as follows. Get on hands and knees or on elbows and knees, on the carpeted floor. (See Figure 3.) While in this position, deepen the spine between the shoulder blades into as much of a hollow as you can. Feel those shoulder blades coming together, touching or almost touching. Now lift that area between the shoulder blades as far upward as possible. You will see the scapular area widening, the shoulder blades coming apart. Do this with much vigor. Get into an energetic rhythm of deepening and lifting the area between the shoulder blades one after the other, going in and out, in and out repeatedly. This exercises the lateral ligaments that will tend to work misplaced and badly positioned vertebral bodies back into normal position, thus unpinching the spinal nerves.

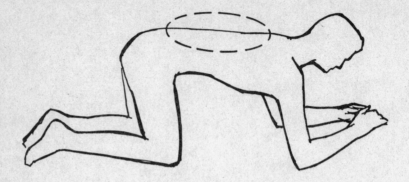

Figure 3

As with the other—and with all—exercises, do this one at anytime during the day but most especially just before retiring.

Unpinching Nerve Pressures in the Small of the Back

This is useful and rewarding for all persons but most beneficial in the immediate sense for those with lumbago, sciatica, sacroiliac problems and other low back discomforts. This one is also done on hands and knees or on elbows and knees, whichever suits better. Now, however, the small of the back is vigorously deepened into as hollow a swayback as possible. (See Figure 4.) Lower the end of the spine, near the tailbone, as far down as you can. Then arch it as much upward as you can. For the mid-spine you lowered and raised the area between the shoulder blades in successive, energetic movements. Here it is done with the area of the low back.

Another way that unpinches nerve pressures in both the mid-spine and lower spine—and a way that is also fun—is to walk around the room on hands and knees. (See Figure 5.) Walk or even run a race on hands and knees. Choose the longest hallway or most spacious room of the house and do some active reconnoitering of the place on hands and knees. For a change of pace, stop on your hands and knees, lower to the elbows and knees, and now do a series of hollowings and archings of the spine with great vigor from this position.

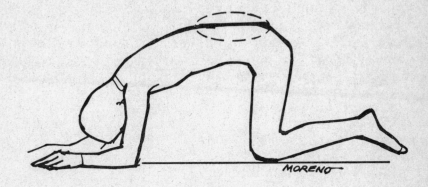

Figure 4

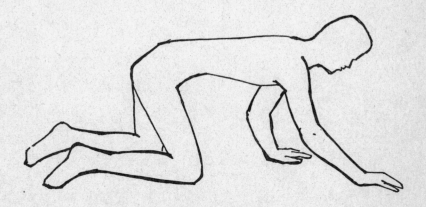

Figure 5

A third way to unpinch spinal nerves and at the same time tend to bring every vertebra into correct juxtaposition with its neighbor is this. Sitting, think of your buttocks and tighten them. (See Figure 6.). Bring those cheeks together tightly until they touch, or almost do, as if holding a pencil between them. Now, with feet flat on the floor, consciously raise the vertebrae headward. Begin by lifting each vertebra in the lower spine off the pelvis, then lift the vertebrae from there to the nape of the neck. Finally lift the segments of the neck toward the top of the head. Feel the elongation of the spine as you do this. Try the same thing while lying on your back. A little of this can go a long way. It may be very tiring. Do some of this before retiring.

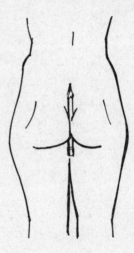

Figure 6

Bursitis Drills and Exercises

Whenever a bursa in your body is inflamed, you have bursitis. The bursa is a kind of little oil-bag to hold down friction at joints. Most bursitis occurs at the shoulder, but tennis players call it a tennis elbow and football players sometimes call it a housemaid's knee. I have found that rest periods *plus* mild stretchings between rest periods helps bursitis of most varieties better than the customary immobilization-diathermy-injections of the medical man.

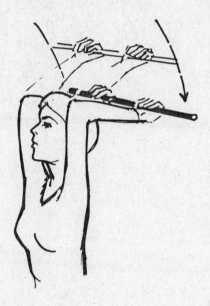

Figure 7

For the most common bursitis problems, those which occur at the shoulders, raise a ruler or cane or broomstick overhead, holding the stick with both hands about eight inches apart. (See Figure 7.) Without lowering the elbows, try to lower the stick to the top of the head. The tendency will be to lower the elbows also, but this must be resisted. As you employ the elbows as "hinges" in this way, the forearms go backward with the stick in your hands and the bursae get mildly stretched. Following a few of these movements, spread the hands that hold the stick to where they are about two feet apart. Now, holding the stick aloft, lower it to the shoulders in back of your head. What you will do is raise the stick overhead, holding it about two feet apart with both hands, then bring it down and rest it on your shoulders *in back of your head.* As you bring the stick down you may feel the need to wiggle it into place behind your head. After a few trials it will come easier, for the bursae will be stretched, and you will be able to bring the stick straight down from overhead to the shoulder rest behind your head.

Another useful way to stretch the bursae is to hang very gingerly from a chinning bar or rafter of loops overhead. The best way is to use loops that fit snugly around the wrists. Let your weight down easily, don't hang there for too long a time at first, repeat this several times a day, especially at bedtime.

For Strengthening and "Un-Paining" Wrists and Ankles

When some people trip over anything they break their ankles instead of breaking the fall with strong ankles. When they fall forward they break their wrists instead of breaking their fall with strong enough wrists to protect them. But anyone who does the drills that follow will almost surely develop strong ankles and wrists.

Hold a broomstick or mopstick in tightly clenched fingers, arm stretched in front of you full length. Gripping the stick firmly, turn it clockwise as far as it will go, then counterclockwise as far as it will go. Do this repeatedly in both directions until the wrist feels a bit tired—which, at first, will be very soon. Now do the same thing with the other hand, arm extended straight out in front of you. Following this, the arm is extended out to the side as you twirl the stick in tightly gripped fingers as far as you can in each direction. Finally do this with the stick straight up overhead. (See Figure 8.) In each position as you twirl the stick you will feel that you exercise muscles way up in the arm near the shoulder joint, but most of all it will exercise and strengthen the wrist area. The eight little carpal bones which are so tightly packed together in that small space will, perhaps for the first time, be expanded and loosened to allow blood nutrition to course through them as the stick in your hand turns in both directions.

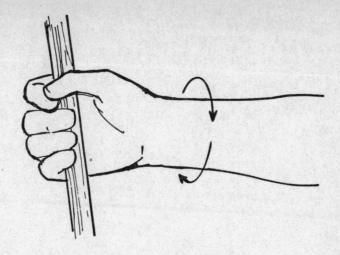

Figure 8

For the ankles, the great need in most persons is to work the tendons of Achilles and strengthen them so that they properly support the ankle area. Standing beside a low stool or chair, place one foot flat on the raised surface or seat of the chair. While being sure that you do not raise the heel, bend forward at the knee as far as you can. (See Figure 9.) To hold the foot down flat while bending the knee far forward you will need to stretch the Achilles tendon. Very quickly you will feel the pull in that tendon. Bring the knee backward to ease the pull on the tendon, then bend it forward again. Do this many times with both feet alternately. In bed, also, while flat on your back, you can exercise and strengthen these tendons by trying to curl your toes upward and headward toward the shinbones.

Another ankle strengthener is this: Stand with feet four inches apart, parallel to each other. Now roll them outward until you are standing on their outer margins. Go back and forth from positions on the flat of your feet to the outside margins of the feet, repeating until tired at the ankles. While on the outside of the feet, if done with enough vigor the inside soles of the feet will almost face each other as the legs bow out.

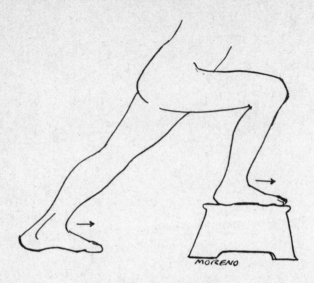

Figure 9

For the sturdy ones, while on the outside edges of the feet try to do some toe-raising. This needs Spartan valor and discipline to do, but the rewards are great.

Finally, stand with feet about six inches apart and bring the toes together in pigeon-toed fashion. While thus pigeon-toed try to raise yourself on the tips of your toes. (See Figure 10.) A few toe-raising efforts while thus pigeon-toed will let the ankles know they are being worked and strengthened.

NOTE: The latter two drills are also excellent for those with varicose veins that give constant pain. Toe-raising while on the edges of the feet, and toe-raising while in pigeon-toed position both tend to lift the valvular areas in the legs that are distended into varicosities.

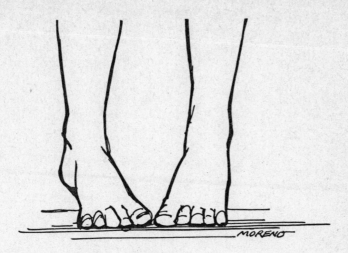

Figure 10

For Varicose Veins

While on the subject of distressing, ballooned varicose veins, the best single activity I know is running backward in a pool of water, lifting the knees high as you run backward. (See Figure 11.) This offers no magic results, unfortunately, but in the matter of varicose veins where nothing significant has ever been devised of a truly helpful nature, this is the best drill I have ever used. Along with the two aforementioned exercises for the ankles (q.v.), the veins will receive some help, although not as much as may be desired. Also, running backward on the sandy beach often proves helpful even without immersion in water.

For Chest Pains and Constricted Feelings at the Breastbone

Here we may be dealing with serious conditions that need a great deal of help. While walking, if you have to stop with chest pains, a helpful natural aid is to touch the palms of your hands behind your back and, while the palms are thus in contact with each other, roll the elbows inward. (See Figure 12.) This opens the chest. It also spreads the ribs apart for better breathing. Best of all it aligns the spine in back of the chest area. Just do this while looking at yourself sideways in the mirror. What a great exercise this is for stooped shoulders! How it straightens the spine, lifts the pectoral areas and strengthens the breast muscles at the same time! Do this for general spine-alignment even if you do not need to do it for chest discomforts.

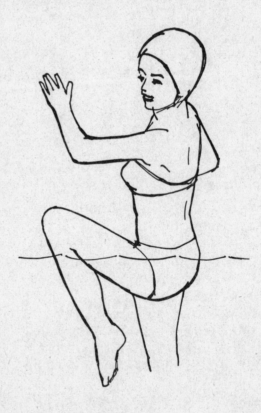

Figure 11

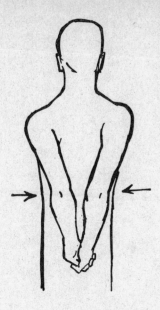

Figure 12

Another drill for this is what I call the Rib-Widener. Standing or sitting, be conscious of your lower ribs and separate them. Bring them apart. (See Figure 13.) Widen them with a vigorous effort. This opens the lower chest space as nothing else can, permits you to use the residual air in the lower lobes of the lungs, and is a reoxygenating exercise that I would have all teachers relay to all the children in the schools.

For Difficult Breathing, Wheezing and Low Oxygenating Capacity

It is not alone pain, as such, which causes discomfort, for when one is embarrassed for breath with every inhalation he is a close rival of anyone with great pain in the discomfort area. If you have to fight for breath, or can hear yourself wheezing as you breathe, read the foregoing Rib-Widener drill and do this with frequency, especially before retiring.

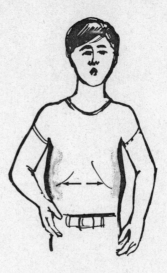

Figure 13

My two favorite exercises for improving the breathing mechanism are simply favorite because they achieve the best results in quickest time. First, lift both arms above the head and pant slightly through parted lips, noting the diaphragm being exercised in and out as you pant. (See Figure 14.) Do this and look at your mid-section, just below the breastbone. With arms aloft and lips parted, do some panting and note the diaphragm working in and out in unison. This is one of the very strongest muscles in the entire body. It has become almost semiparalyzed from disuse, because we are shallow breathers and do not work this muscle to inhale and exhale with the lower lobes. By doing this diaphragmatic drill you will strengthen the diaphragm and breathe again as the baby does—the stomach going in and out with each breath. This one drill alone is worth the effort of going to China to learn. It spells breath and life.

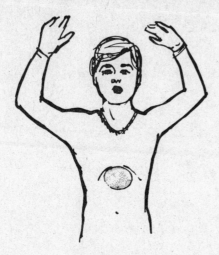

Figure 14

The second favorite reoxygenating drill is also valuable beyond calculation. It is the one best way I know to make our entire breathing apparatus strong. And it is incredibly easy. Merely count twice as long exhaling as you can count inhaling. While walking, get into the habit of taking in your breath to, say, the count of four, and then letting the breath out to the count of eight. Or six and twelve. Or seven and fourteen. Whatever. Just count twice as long on the exhalation as on the inhalation. This forces the muscles to strengthen toward the last of each exhaling count—just notice it yourself. In a short time your breathing mechanism will improve, you will suffer fewer colds, your wheezing and difficult gasping for breath will be memories of the past.

For Arriving at the Correct Posture for YOU

There is no such thing as "a correct posture." It is different for different persons. What is the exactly correct posture for you may not be correct for anyone else on earth. It depends upon your individual weight, your height, your bone structure, the "architecture" of your framework. Thus the old West Point ideal of "chest up, chin in, spine stiff" is sadly ridiculous to anyone who has really studied human structure.

But there is a way to ascertain *your* correct posture. A perfectly easy way, a perfect way, a way that is foolproof and fits your own individual needs, not a way that fits any masses as "the correct posture."

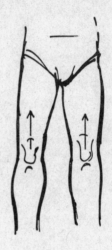

Figure 15

Stand flat on both feet, arms hanging at sides, feet parallel and about four inches apart. Now try to raise your little toes, all except the great toe, by curling them upward while standing flat on your feet. In doing this you automatically find the right stance on those feet of yours, for you will notice the weight shifting to a new position as your toes curl upward. Following this you do these things in order. Tighten the buttocks. Bring them smartly together to where they almost touch. Lift the kneecaps with vigor up toward the pelvis (Figure 15) drop your shoulders, then be conscious of flattening your shoulder blades against the backbone. (See Figure 16.) You will be surprised to find that you hardly knew your shoulder blades have been sticking out like angel's wings. From this point all you need do is endeavor to lift the head off the shoulders in a spine-lengthening effort centered in the neck and—presto! you have found the correct posture. This is the correct one for you! Individually yours. Since postural faults bring many pains and discomforts in their wake, learning how to realize your own true postural position is to learn how to avoid pains and discomforts ahead.

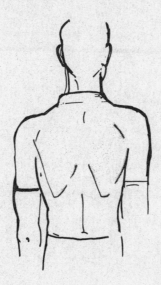

Figure 16

For Recurring Sacroiliac Pains

Some people have trouble in their sacroiliac joints all their lives. It is difficult to reach these joints specifically with any one exercise. But after working on this for a while I have devised a drill that specifically helps these articulations. Added to the others for the low back and the mid spine, what follows should greatly strengthen and relieve pains in the sacroiliac joints.

Stand on flat feet, with feet together. Raising the right foot, place the ankle on the opposite leg, resting the right ankle just above the left kneecap. While thus standing on one foot, the left one, swing the right bent knee outward toward the right tip. (See Figure 17.) Swing it outward with enough vigor to feel it in the backbone. Where you will feel the effect of the outward swing will be exactly at the saroiliac joint.

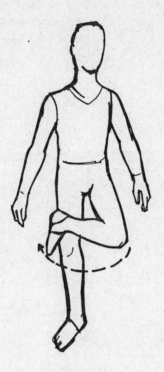

Figure 17

Now raise the left foot and place the left ankle above the kneecap of the right leg. Maintaining your balance on one foot as best you can, bring the left bent leg outward and backward as far as you can. Feel it in the backbone, just to the side of the last vertebra.

Alternate the move, switching from right to left with speed and vigor. Some people say that they can best maintain balance on one foot if they touch the palms of their hands in front of the chest in a praying position and fix their gaze on a single spot directly in front. This appears to stabilize them. However you balance on one foot, by swinging out the bent knee of one leg after another (while the ankle of that bent leg rests on the opposite thigh) you will reach and strengthen the sacroiliac articulations.

For a General "Un-Paining" of Hurting Joints

In my entire career I have never seen or devised anything better than *walking on hands and feet* for providing elasticity and a tune-up for all the joints of the body.

In another book, *Doctor Morrison's Miracle Body Tune-Up for Rejuvenated Health,* I have called this The Primordial Walk. I cannot improve on the name. It is the way I envision the manner of locomotion way back in primordial times. You will note above that is says "walking on hands and feet." Not on hands and knees, but *feet.* (See Figure 18.) This stretches, and exercises, and provides suppleness to all muscles, ligaments, cartilages, tendons and everything else in the body I can think of.

If starting this in middle age or later, it can be hard to take. I advise a mere step or two on hands and feet at first. The Primordial Walk, however, has the capability of building strength into the body rapidly. In a few days you will want to walk around the room on hands and feet. After such a walk you won't be satisfied with less than a big romp on the lawn or the back yard on hands and feet. When you train your children or teenagers to do this, you'll find they can plunge into vigorous Primordial Walks at once, then keep it up forever with great benefits to their pain-free future.

In the beginning, when walking on hands and feet, do not turn your head up and strain the neck thereby. Keep the neck elongated in the manner of a four-legged animal grazing, with head down. Also, I hope you can manage to do the Primordial Walk with bare feet touching the soil or grass and thus contacting Mother Earth. This is one exercise that is an invigorator in the morning but may be overstimulating when done at bedtime.

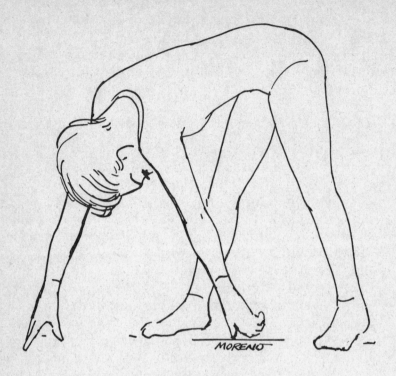

Figure 18

Specifically for Hurting Knees and Elbows

By far the majority of knee pains I have encountered were the result of a backward-misplaced tibia, or shin-bone. I have checked this with other doctors, and all were surprised about it. But when the patient was made to sit on a high table, with the hurting knee on the level of the doctor's chest, and the doctor snapped the back-slipped tibial bone forward, the patient could at once get off the table and walk without pain.

One diagnostic sign is this: If the knee hurts more on descending than on ascending a staircase, the tibia probably has been yanked out of position. The head of the tibia, which is just below the knee in what is called the popliteal area, needs to be moved forward because some strain or fall has caused it to be jerked backward. A runner, for example, on lunging forward in a footrace when the starter says "Go!" puts a fearful strain on the tibia and can cause it to come out of position. On replacing the bone for professional runners, their relief and cessation of pain was immediate.

To get this done at home, lie on the back and place a small pillow or towel rolled into a cylinder in that popliteal area just back of the knee. Bend the knee around the pillow or towel-roll. Wedge it tightly into the bend of the knee right behind the kneecap. Now hold the ankle and gently bring the foot toward the buttock on that side. The towel-roll under the knee will force an expansion of the space, it will stretch the area, it will tend to bring the head of the tibia backward into correct position. Often you will hear a small "click" as the tibial bone returns to normal position.

For the elbow, place a rolled towel into the bend of the elbow and gently bring the wrist on that side back toward the shoulder, using the cylindrical roll in the bend of the elbow as a fulcrum to stretch the parts wider. Even a rolling pin in the crook of the elbow will do the trick. Cover the rolling pin with a towel and place it in the bend of the elbow, then stretch the elbow joint by bringing the wrist on the affected side toward the shoulder. This is well done at bedtime, and it helps most especially after a relaxing *Neutral Bath* (q.v.).

For Eyestrain from Television Viewing

When the head aches and the eyes burn or hurt after viewing television for a long time, it is time to learn a small lesson. The muscles of the eyes get overstrained when one is seated too close to the TV set. The rule has been worked out and should be widely broadcast. It is this.

Sit one foot away from the set for every inch of screen size.

If you have a 23-inch screen, for example, you should sit a distance of 23 feet from the set. Any closer than this and your eye muscles unconsciously tense, overwork, tend toward spasms. The screen size is measured diagonally. If your living room size does not permit your sitting so far away from the set, the obvious solution is to get a smaller set. Modern TV sets with small screen size are even sharper and clearer than large ones.

For Pains in the Feet and Legs from Flat Feet

Two wonderful exercises are available to rework fallen arch bones upward into correct position. One is that of rolling on an old-fashioned rolling pin. Stand with both feet on a rolling pin, preferably after a warm foot bath, and hold on to chairs or dressers on each side to prevent falling. Now roll back and forth on the rolling pin, thus lifting the collapsed arch bones back to their normal situs. (See Figure 19.) Do this with both feet on the rolling pin even if only one foot needs the treatment; or else a structural imbalance of the body may result. And do this at bedtime for sure. The reason is that after this treatment of lifting the seven tarsal bones into an arch, it is best to immediately go to bed and take your weight off your feet instead of walking and pounding the lifted bones down again.

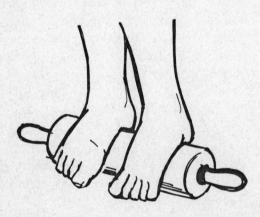

Figure 19

The other foot exercise of great merit, already mentioned, is the pidgeon-toed toe-raising drill. (See Figure 10.) Assume a pidgeon-toed position by pointing your toes inward toward each other. Now merely go up and down on your toes until you are tired. Do this at bedtime especially. It usually works wonders in restoring the arches and general contours of your feet.

Chapter Thirty-Two

Putting the Whole Book Together

As the author, I must assume that you have read this book—every chapter of it.

Certain of the *researches* must have "caught" you, and will forever stay with you.

What are the highlights, the luminous points of the book that you will want to remember? What are the new and provocative researches in the book that you will want to talk to your friends about?

Well, in order that "he who runs may read," here follow in quick, pithy *remembering sentences* the central meaty points of what have gone before. Not all of them, to be sure, for that would equal a full rewriting of the book and your complete rereading of it. But I would fondly hope that you do just that— reread all the *chapters* time and again. For now, however, as quick reminders of what has gone before, ready—set—go!

*Don't overfluidize your cells and system but drink only in answer to an actual thirst signal; otherwise, whatever your drink may be, it will not fill a physiological need of your body.

*Do not allow drinks or foods to enter your mouth that are too hot to touch with bare hands, or are too hot to dip your fingers into.

*Remember that resting on your back causes the organs to be upside down, so to speak, so give yourself an occasional *good* rest by lying face down with the head hanging over the edge of the bed slightly lower than the rest of the body.

*If constipated, think of assuming a squat position that enables the descending colon and rectum to lengthen, or tip the toilet seat up in front and down in back.

*If you feel debilitated and you are using electric blankets for nightly warmth, consider that whenever you artificially induce warmth that your own body should be generating you are robbing your own organism of one of its functions, and weakening it thereby.

*If you believe that, as the Bible has it, "the life is in the blood," then you know that all the blood donor's tendencies and weaknesses may be transferred with his blood to the one who gets the transfusion; so consider requesting normal saline solutions for any transfusions, you may need. Saline solutions can start up the body's own blood-manufacturing apparatus, and produce for you your own type of blood instead of a stranger's. Another way is to give a pint of your own blood say three weeks before your scheduled surgery, thus storing your individual blood sample for use in case of need.

*Despite feeling warm and tingling with health after a cold plunge, consider that this is a neurological shock and may do eventual harm.

*Foreign growths or lumps in the female breast may be seen under transilluminating lights in a dark closet, after which a program of unpinching nerve pressures to the breast area, plus a fast which forces the body to consume its own resident protein may, in many cases, absorb the breast lumps without recourse to mastectomy.

*Since constant chewing of gum causes constant manufacture and swallowing of saliva, this needlessly spurs the production of an enzyme needed in starch digestion and exhausts the salivary glands; therefore those who continually chew gum can bring on their own digestive problems.

*Human exercise should be done, preferably, using both sides of the body equally, as is true of rowing, throwing volleyballs, bicycling, swimming, running, skating; and in illness we recommend drills that are superior to unilateral exercises such as golf or bowling which tend to distort the body structure one-sidedly.

*Since elderly people have memory lapses from insufficient blood supply (and oxygen) to tiny brain vessels, to have them rest in bed boosted *up* on pillows prevents further the circulation of blood, and this needs a rethink and change from the current gravitational up-flow on high pillows to a possible down-flow of blood that may more easily reach their poorly oxygenated cranial vessesls.

*An overconsumption of proteins causes proteins to decompose in human intestines and change into three smelly acids, all of which make human stools foul and odorous; thus toothbrushes, towels and such cleaning aids might better be hung inside cabinets where the foul and odor-bearing bacteria in bathrooms do not enter the bristles or towels.

*From the human lifestyle of living upright, against gravity, people tend toward a round-shouldered or hump-backed condition in their upper spine, and this presses on nerves to the stomach and digestive organs; thus, the exercise herein named "Dowager's Hump" can unpinch vertebral nerve pressures in this area and help conditions of dyspepsia, etc.

*Telling people to take an after-dinner stroll to "walk down their dinner" is ridiculous and physiologically wrong, for after a meal the blood is needed in the digestive organs and walking pulls some of the blood away to the muscles of locomotion—therefore, watch the animals and note how they instinctively curl up and nap after eating.

*Hunting cures for the common cold will always be unfulfilling research because *the cold itself is the cure;* for it is nature's way of opening the eliminative channels to permit outflow of accumulated toxic debris, sneezing out the waste products, or coughing them up, or burning them up through fevers, etc.

*Eating fruit skins "because they contain the best vitamins and minerals" may be so much flapdoodle because it appears that the body manufactures no enzymes strong enough to break them down to their normal end-products of digestion, which is why we sometimes see undigested tomato skins in the stools. Skins are impermeable and made to keep the nutrients inside, not to themselves be eaten.

*Since sunbathing can and does cause burning of the skin

that may produce cancer, it is well to know that when the sun's rays are slanted before ten in the morning and after four in the afternoon (when your shadow is longer than you are tall) there is no danger to the human being and one can sunbathe with impunity.

*Disregarding the all-too-common advice to consume high protein diets may be the first step toward better health, for the body is strictly limited in how much protein it can utilize, and so any excess protein is toxin-building and health-destroying in the human body.

*Because the body mends its damaged cells during quiet sleep and what you gain at bedtime you tend to retain during bedtime, the best of all exercise times is at night, just before retiring.

*People who eat good and organically grown and properly combined food but still remain sick should realize that the potential value of any food is not its actual value, that it must first be appropriated and utilized, and that nerve pressures to the digestive organs may interfere with the flow of "digesting power" to those organs.

*The greatest benefits from exercises inevitably flow from doing exercise movements in a horizontal position, for then the heart does not need to pump blood uphill and arteries do not need to be dilated and strained.

*Since milk is a protein food, and the body has no provision for utilizing protein except when it is chewed (not drunk), you should reconsider your need for drinking milk.

*Since man is a primate, and the natural food of the primate is almost exclusively fruits, when you are baffled about your ailment, and the doctors are also baffled, go the Primate Diet of fruits for a week and the body, thus given a rest, will nearly always sort out the trouble and tend to heal itself.

*Even those with a history of coronary occlusion should do some exercise for the heart, and *especially* these cardiac cripples need exercises within their capacity to do, because when the pulse-rate goes to 100 or over nature tends to "build in" small auxiliary vessels. These auxiliary vessels serve the stricken heart area that is cut off from blood nutrition by the sludge-filled artery.

*Aristotle's method of using geometric figures and patterns to expand the memory and make new brain cells pop ought to be universally taught and used, especially by students before a difficult examination, by adults entering into complicated contract talks, etc.

*With our substandard ecological conditions it is vital to "make do" with what oxygen is available under our polluted sky canopy, and these researches afford simple means of both strengthening the breathing apparatus and making better use, through better oxygenation, of the available air.

*Careful objective research indicates that the body mechanically gets out of adjustment more often than it gets chemically imbalanced; that faulty body mechanics can cause nerve pressures with ensuing chemistry dysfunctions, but not the other way around; that we are born with a complete chemical factory, able to make all the insulin, adrenalin, pepsin, cortisone and the rest that we need, but we are not born with a complete mechanical equipment, for at birth we cannot even sit up, much less walk, run, heave, lug, strain—and when we adjust to these strains we get out of adjustment, and no machine that is out of adjustment can be *reasonably* expected to work right; thus, mechanical faults need first attention.

*Since we turn and twist the neck more often than other parts of the body, and nerves traversing the neck freed Life Power to all organs below, this technique of easily self-helping the neck out of nerve pressures by lifting the head off the shoulders, and turning the head while lifting, is of greatest importance and benefit in the realm of scientifically unpinching pinched nerves and restoring real *natural* health.

*By exercising the muscles of side vision through these peripheral drills, the out-of-round eyes are frequently returned to normal roundness and eye problems, even migraine headaches referable to the eyes, may vanish.

*The diets for all seasons meet a variety of conditions: for losing weight naturally and effectively; for strengthening a weak heart; for normalizing the kidneys and urinary bladder; for naturally helping asthma and emphysema; for soothing and nourishing the nervous system; even a compromise diet for those who feel they cannot follow diets.

*Since all people wish to live a long time if only the years ahead could be pain-free years, this collection of the very best drills and exercises in all the known healing arts is *specifically* designed to strengthen weak body parts, and to take pains away from joints, muscles, tendons, ligaments, pinched nerves and aching organs, and can enable anyone, with minimal effort, to live a relatively effective and pain-free life.

Index